Teaching Atlas of Hand Radiology

S. Gilani & B.K. Wignall

W.B. Saunders Company Ltd
London · Philadelphia · Toronto
Sydney · Tokyo

W.B. Saunders 24–28 Oval Road
Company Ltd   London NW1 7DX, UK

The Curtis Center
Independence Square West
Philadelphia, PA 19106–3399, USA

Harcourt Brace
& Company
55 Horner Avenue
Toronto, Ontario M8Z 4X6, Canada

Harcourt Brace & Company, Australia
30–52 Smidmore Street
Marrickville, NSW 2204, Australia

Harcourt Brace, Japan
Ichibancho Central Building,
22–1 Ichibancho
Chiyoda-ku, Tokyo 102, Japan

A catalogue record for this book is available from the British Library

ISBN 0–7020–1731–0

Typeset by Fakenham Photosetting Ltd, Fakenham, Norfolk
Printed and bound in Great Britain by
The University Press, Cambridge

Contents

Preface

Many diseases affect the hand. Some are limited to the hand but more commonly, they are included in a more widespread disorder of the bones and joints, or part of a disorder primarily of other systems. Hence, examination of the hand both clinically and radiographically is frequently of help in diagnosis.

Radiography of the hand may also be of use to assess the progress of diseases their response to treatment. This depends on the changes demonstrated often being representative of skeletal abnormalities at other sites.

Additionally, hand radiographs are technically simple to produce showing fine structural details with minimal radiation exposure to the patient.

The authors who are involved in both undergraduate and postgraduate teaching, have presented each case in an identical way using easily understood terms with a minimum of radiological jargon:–

■ CLINICAL FEATURES PLUS RADIOGRAPHY
   To include age, sex and ethnic origin.

■ RADIOGRAPHIC OBSERVATIONS
   Anatomic site and distribution of lesion, whether bone, synovial, joint or soft tissue primarily involved.

   Characteristics of lesion – particularly to differentiate benign or malignant: acute from chronic.

■ DIAGNOSTIC POSSIBILITIES
   Including differential where relevant and diseases classification.

■ EXPLANATORY NOTES
   Mainly on radiographic appearance at other sites and appropriate further imaging techniques and other investigations.

This layout is intended to promote a systematic, disciplined approach and to emphasise that individual signs are not considered in isolation when arriving at a differential diagnosis.

The largely pictorial content of the Atlas will also assist with pattern recognition, which is equally important in radiological diagnosis. The self assessment format is a well established method of promoting enforcement of learning. The contents are easily assimiable.

The amount of text is kept to a minimum and because an Atlas cannot be comprehensive, it should be used in conjunction with one of the several text books of skeletal radiology; a short list of recommended text books for reference is included.

The Atlas is produced primarily for those preparing for postgraduate qualifications in Radiology, Medicine and Surgery. In addition, the Atlas may prove useful to final year medical students, general practitioners, orthopaedic surgeons and rheumatologists with an interest in diseases involving bones and joints.

S. Gilani
B.K. Wignall

Acknowledgements

The authors are extremely indebted for the loan of some radiographs from colleagues at the following hospitals - Hillingdon, St Thomas', Royal National Orthopaedic, St Mary's (London) and Manchester Royal Infirmary.

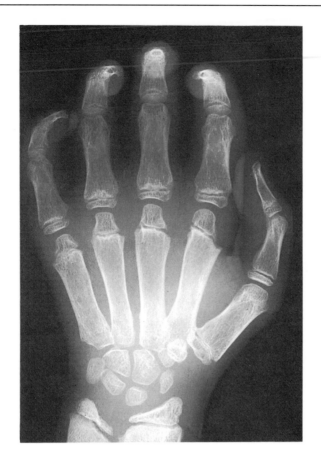

Relevant clinical features

■ Corneal opacities.
■ Short stature.
■ Coarse facial features, large tongue.
■ Mentally retarded.

CASE 1

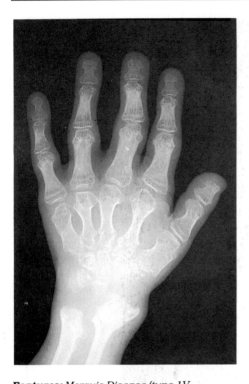

Observations

- Conical shape of metacarpals, broad distal part and narrow base.
- Radius and ulna tipping towards each other.
- Angulation and wavy contour of the metaphyses.
- Expansion of bone with thinning of the cortex.

Features: *Morquio Disease (type 1V mucopolysaccharidosis). Irregular small carpals. Short metacarpals with irregular heads and bases. Cupped irregular articular surfaces of radius and ulna. Children not usually mentally retarded. Facial features normal.*

Diagnosis

MUCOPOLYSACCHARIDOSIS: type 1 (Hurler syndrome syn. Gargoyle).

Notes

Skeletal survey should be performed to differentiate between the different types of dwarfism/congenital dysplasias. In Hurler syndrome multiple bony abnormalities include large thick skull vault with J-shaped sella. Flaring of ilia with shallow acetabulae and fragmentation of femoral capital epiphyses, paddle-shaped ribs, hypoplasia of one or more vertebral bodies with an anterior beak-like protrusion on their inferior aspects. An inherited (autosomal recessive) condition confirmed by the genetic defect and the particular mucopolysaccharide in the urine. Children usually die within first year. Insert shows features of mucopolysaccharidosis is type 1V. Types 1 and 1V are the commonest in this group.

2

CASE 2: Girl aged 14 years

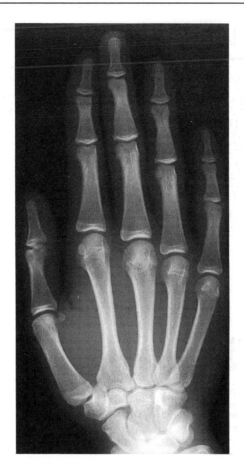

Relevant clinical features
- Tall thin girl.
- Hypermobile joints.
- Heart murmur.

CASE 2

Metacarpal index =

$$\Sigma \left(\frac{\text{Length of matacarpal shaft}}{\text{Width}} \right) / 4$$

Metacarpal index = 9.12

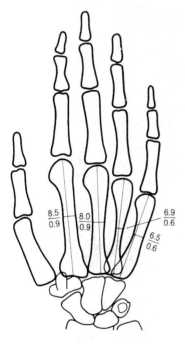

Observations

■ Long slender tubular bones (metacarpal index >9). (Normal range 5.4–7.9) Abnormal >8.4

Diagnosis

ARACHNODACTYLY: Marfan's syndrome. Hereditary collagen disorder.

Notes

Autosomal dominant. Arachnodactyly can occur in the absence of Marfan's syndrome:

■ Eyes: bilateral lens dislocation.

■ Cardiovascular system: mitral incompetence, atrial septal defect, aortic dilatation with dissecting aneurysms.

■ Bones: posterior scalloping of vertebral bodies, scoliosis, sternal deformity and arched palate.

CASE 3: Female aged 40 years

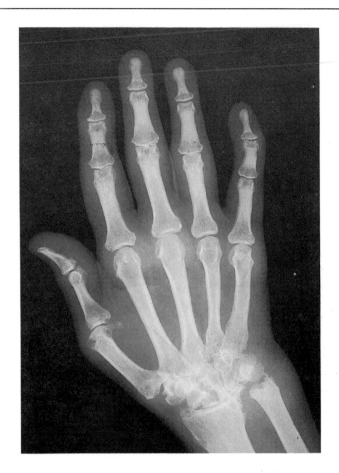

Relevant clinical features

■ For past 5 years recurrent morning stiffness lasting 20 mins.

■ Symmetrical swelling and pain involving the MCP joint of the index, middle and little fingers.

■ Similar symptoms in MTP joints of the feet and wrist.

■ Recent deformity of middle, index, MCP joints left hand.

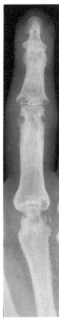

Observations

- Multiple defects (erosions) at margins of MCP joints and radioulnar joint.
- More extensive cyst-like erosions of ulnar styloid process and at bases of proximal phalanges of index and middle fingers.
- Soft tissue swelling around MCP and wrist joints.
- Narrowing of MCP and carpal joints.
- Subluxation of index and middle MCP joints with ulna deviation of fingers.
- Reduction in bone density adjacent to joint margins (juxta-articular osteoporosis).

Features: Advanced marginal erosions (some corticated) in MCP and PIP joints.

Diagnosis

RHEUMATOID ARTHRITIS: collagen disease with associated inflammatory polyarthropathy.

Differential diagnosis

PSORIATIC ARTHROPATHY: (see *Case 29*) mainly DIP involvement. No osteoporosis. Associated skin rash and nail changes.

GOUT: (see *Case 4*) asymmetrical soft-tissue masses, no osteoporosis juxta-articular erosions.

Notes

More common in females. Age of onset variable, 40–60 years. Radiographic changes may never occur and usually presents only after 2–3 months of symptoms (see *Case 92*).

- Soft tissue swelling: symmetrical; around joints due to effusions.
- Erosions: at joint margins. Characteristic early radiographic change. Usually bilaterally at MTP joints, MCP joints of index, middle fingers, wrist and ulnar styloids.
- Hand PIP joints less commonly involved. DIP joints virtually spared.

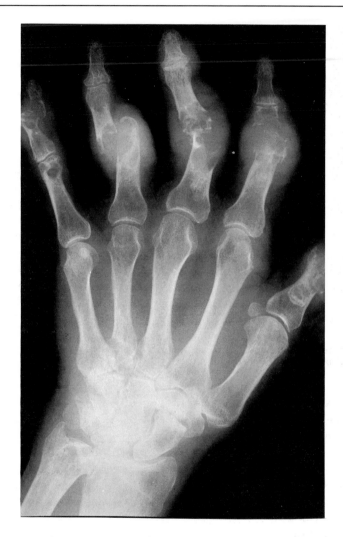

Relevant clinical features

- Painful joints.
- Associated soft-tissue swelling.
- Skin red and inflamed.

CASE 4

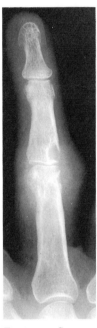

Observations

■ Asymmetrical soft-tissue swellings around many IP joints.

■ Multiple asymmetrical punched-out erosions at the joint margins and extending along the cortex of the shafts involving ring finger, PIP joint, middle and little fingers DIP joints and the IP joints of index finger.

■ Cyst-like subchondral lesions in head of thumb, index, and proximal phalanx.

■ Loss of bone density around affected joints.

Features: Same patient ring finger, right hand, showing very large intraosseous tophi around PIP joint.

Diagnosis

GOUT: metabolic deposition arthropathy.

Differential diagnosis

RHEUMATOID ARTHRITIS: (see *Case 3*).   PSORIATIC ARTHROPATHY: (see *Case 29*).

Notes

Deposition of urates in synovium causes acutely painful hot joints. Male/female ratio 20 : 1. Commoner over 40 years. X-ray changes not seen until ⩾6 years after first attack. Radiographic changes:

■ Erosions: start near joint margins, sharply marginated, extend along cortex of shaft rather than articular surfaces. Cartilage destruction late.

■ Soft-tissue swelling: due to deposition of synovial urate crystal aggregates (tophi) may be associated with hot shiny red skin and may calcify.

■ Joint space narrowing: due to cartilage destruction.

■ Intraosseous tophi: causes cyst-like widening of metaphyses.

■ Lack of osteoporosis.

■ Distribution: commonly involves one joint hallus MTP joint (commonest sight), hands, wrists, knees, elbows, SI joints and spine.

■ Complications: ischaemic necrosis femoral and humeral heads. Atlantoaxial subluxation.

CASE 5: Adult male

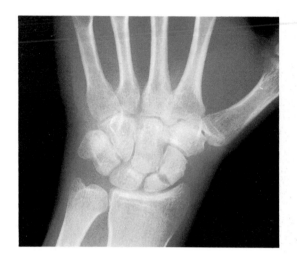

Relevant clinical features

■ Fell on outstretched hand.

CASE 5

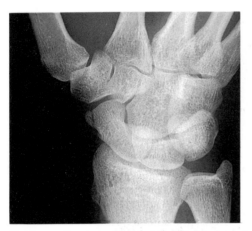

Features: *Fracture of the scaphoid tubercle: unites satisfactorily in thumb spica cast. Blood supply via separate branch of radial artery.*

Observations

■ Low density line through waist of scaphoid with separation of fragments.

Diagnosis

FRACTURED WAIST OF SCAPHOID.

Notes

Forced dorsiflexion causes compression of scaphoid between capitate and radius. Fracture commonest through the waist (70%) at the attachment of the radioscaphocapitate ligamentous sling which passes through the waist of the scaphoid. Can occur in the tubercle (10%) (see inset) and proximal pole (20%). Untreated fractures through the waist or proximal pole may lead to delayed union, non-union or ischaemic necrosis of proximal fragment. Fracture line may not be visible at time of injury. In case of clinical doubt, immediate treatment should be instituted and repeat radiography advised after 10 days. Oblique views of scaphoid must be included.

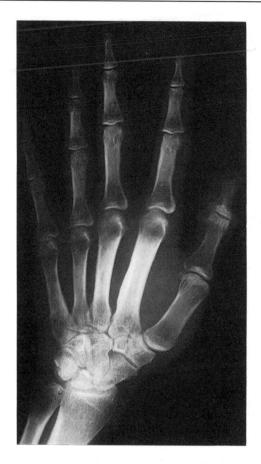

Relevant clinical features
- Muscular weakness, long-standing pains in the arms and legs.
- Waddling gait.

CASE 6

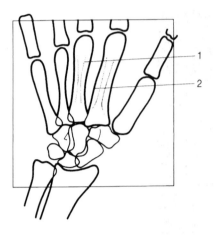

Observations
■ Diaphyseal cortical thickening (particularly endosteal) of index and middle metacarpals and distal radius.

Diagnosis
PROGRESSIVE DIAPHYSEAL DYSPLASIA: (syn. Engelmann–Camurati disease) Hereditary first-degree bone dysplasia.

Differential diagnosis
PAGETS DISEASE: (see *Case 18*) extends to subarticular location, older age group.

CORTICAL HYPEROSTOSIS: (Van Buchem's) generalised condition particularly affecting face and mandible.

FIBROUS DYSPLASIA: (see *Case 58*) asymmetrical involvement.

OSTEOPETROSIS: (see *Case 30*) all bones involved, fractures common.

Notes
Autosomal dominant inheritance. Usual onset 4–12 years. Muscular weakness due to underdevelopment. Usually involves diaphyses of long bones with endosteal and periosteal new bone formation and obliteration of marrow cavities. May involve base of skull. Flat bones rarely involved.

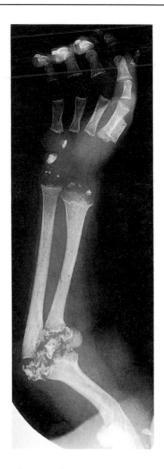

Relevant clinical features

■ Microcephaly.

■ Short limbs.

CASE 7

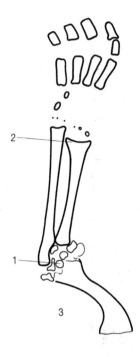

Observations

■ Multiple discrete densities, some punctate, in the region of the carpus and elbow joint, due to calcification.

■ Irregular metaphyses.

■ Shortened humerus.

Diagnosis

CHONDRODYSTROPHIA CALCIFICANS CONGENITA: epiphyseal dysplasia punctata; congenital bone dysplasia.

Notes

There are two types. The above type has *autosomal recessive* inheritance; it is a lethal condition (infants die in first year), with mental retardation, microcephaly, cataracts. The other type (Conradi–Hunermann) has *autosomal dominant* inheritance with normal life expectancy. The metaphyses are normal. In both types there may also be calcification and deformity of lumbar vertebral bodies.

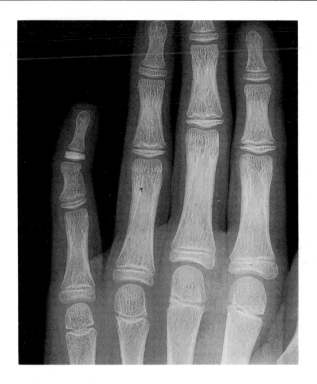

Relevant clinical features
- Mentally retarded.
- Small.
- Slanted palpebral fissures.

CASE 8

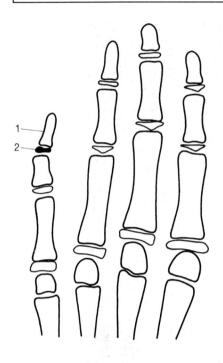

Observations
■ Short curved (i.e. clinodactyly) little finger due to hypoplasia of middle phalanx.
■ Dense epiphysis of terminal phalanx.
■ Bone age 13 years, i.e. delayed maturation.

Diagnosis
DOWN'S SYNDROME: chromosomal abnormality; trisomy 21.

Notes
Above changes seen in 50% of patients. Other changes which may occur are:

■ Pelvis: most commonly abnormal. Wide flared ilia with reduced acetabular angle.
■ Skull and facial bones: small facial bones and sinuses with hypotelorism. Small thin cranium.
■ Thoracic and vertebral abnormalities: squaring of vertebral bodies. Atlantoaxial subluxation. Multiple manubrial ossification centres. Eleven pairs of ribs.
■ Cardiac and vascular abnormalities: congenital heart disease (especially atrioventricular canal defect and ventral septal defect), dextrocardia and aberrant right subclavian artery.
■ Gastrointestinal abnormalities: duodenal atresia and Hirschsprung's disease, and tracheoesophageal fistula.

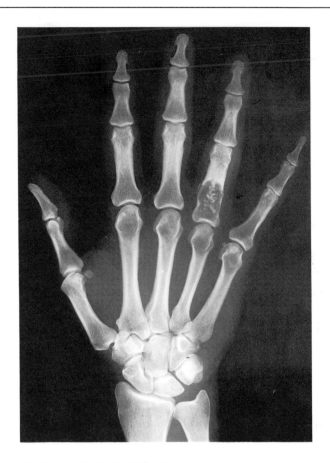

Relevant clinical features
■ Sudden onset of pain in ring finger.

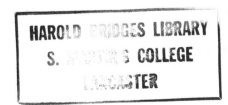

CASE 9

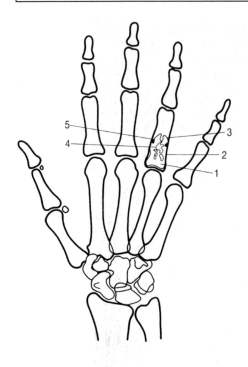

Observations
- Well-defined low density lesion in proximal phalanx of ring finger.
- Bone expanded, cortex well demarcated.
- Inner margin scalloped 'endosteal scalloping'.
- Densities in lesion due to calcification.
- Low-density line through cortex is a fracture.

Diagnosis
ENCHONDROMA: benign cartilaginous tumour.

Notes
Commonly solitary lesion, arising from cartilage rest, situated in medullary cavity. Grows slowly. Often presents as a pathological fracture. Age range 20–50 years. 50% involve short tubular bones of the hand. As tumour cartilaginous origin, few flecks to extensive amorphous calcification common finding. Sarcomatous change rare. Responds well (i.e. no recurrence) to curettage.

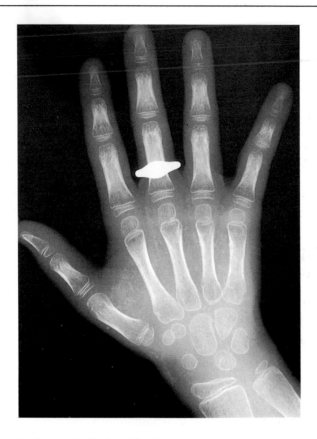

Relevant clinical features
- Rash.
- Fatigue.
- Weakness and pain affecting shoulder muscles.

CASE 10

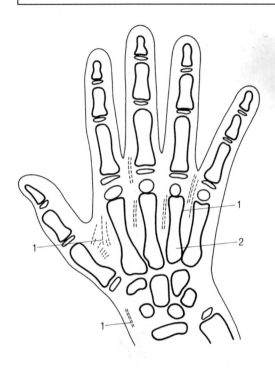

Observations

■ Fine linear densities in the soft tissues, i.e. calcification in both subcutaneous tissue and muscle and follows fascial planes.

■ Osteoporosis due to disuse.

■ Bones otherwise normal.

Diagnosis

DERMATOMYOSITIS: rare collagen disease of unknown aetiology.

Differential diagnosis

SCLERODERMA: skin changes may be identical.

Notes

Commoner in females and may occur in children. Usually involves muscles of neck, shoulders and pelvis, leading to atrophy, fibrosis, calcification and joint contractures. Skin changes, if present, similar to scleroderma. Disuse and steroid therapy leads to osteoporosis. Terminal phalanges of fingers may be small and pointed. Oesophageal motility disorders and pulmonary fibrosis may occur. In adults there is a high incidence of malignant disease, particularly carcinoma of breast and ovary.

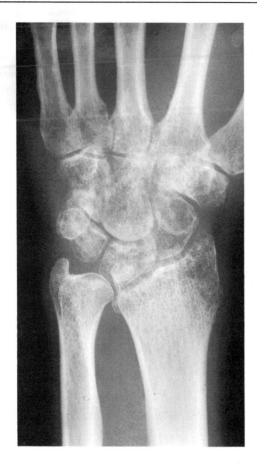

Relevant clinical features
- Intense wrist pain.
- Overlying skin smooth, shiny.
- Fell on hand 1 month previously.

CASE 11

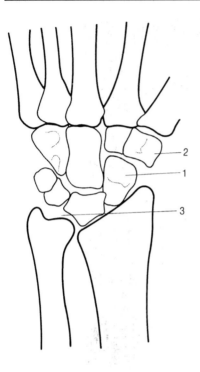

Observations
■ Marked but patchy reduced density of carpal bones, distal radius and ulna.
■ Cortices intact.
■ Joints not affected.

Diagnosis
REFLEX SYMPATHETIC DYSTROPHY SYNDROME (i.e. SUDECK'S ATROPHY).

Notes
Rare condition – usually as a result of a fracture, but may follow trivial trauma as in this case. Represents an extreme type of post traumatic osteoporosis which is associated with skin changes, soft-tissue swelling and severe pain. Symptoms resolve after 6 months. Aetiology unknown.

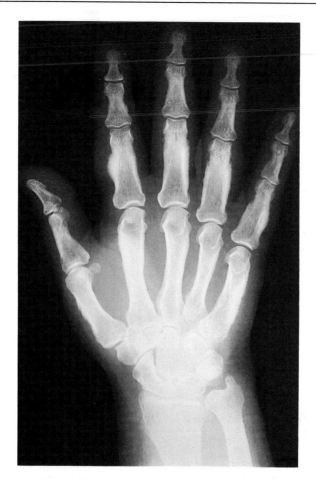

Relevant clinical features
- Previous thyroid ablation by ^{131}I radioactive iodine.
- Soft-tissue swelling over the hands.

CASE 12

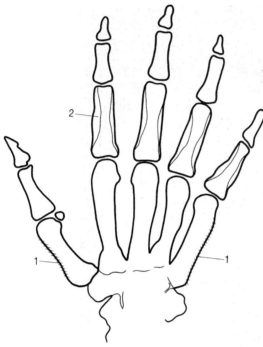

Observations
■ Vertical spiculated and feathery dense bone along shafts of metacarpals and proximal phalanges due to periosteal reaction.
■ Produces cortical thickening in proximal phalanges.

Diagnosis
THYROID ACROPACHY: unknown cause.

Differential diagnosis
HYPERTROPHIC OSTEOARTHROPATHY (HOA): (see *Case 33*) periosteal new bone is parallel to shafts. Pachydermoperiostitis (see *Case 36*).

Notes
More common in males. Usually euthyroid or hypothyroid. Mainly in proximal phalanges of hands. Less common in feet and uncommon in distal ends of forearms and legs. Present years after thyroidectomy or radioisotope therapy for thyrotoxicosis. Extremities swollen or clubbed. Exophthalmos and pretibial myxodema usually present.

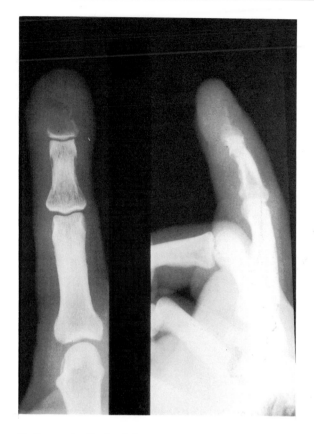

Relevant clinical features
■ Paronychia with acutely painful and swollen distal pulp of index finger.
■ Two-week history.

CASE 13

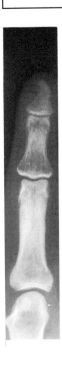

Observations
- Destructive lesion involving terminal phalanx.
- Cortex not visualised.
- Soft-tissue swelling.
- Note: partial reossification after 3 weeks of antibiotic treatment.

Diagnosis
ACUTE PYOGENIC OSTEOMYELITIS: secondary to local soft-tissue infection.

Differential diagnosis
HAEMATOGENOUS INFECTION (see *Case 17*).

Notes
Finger infection commonly due to predisposing local factors, e.g. compound fractures, puncture wounds, bites, burns, individuals with loss of sensation due to syringomyelia and congenital indifference to pain. Soft-tissue swelling precedes bone changes for up to 2 weeks. Radionuclide bone scan should be used to detect the nidus.

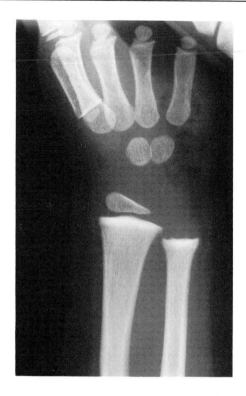

Relevant clinical features
■ Recurrent abdominal pain and vomiting.

CASE 14

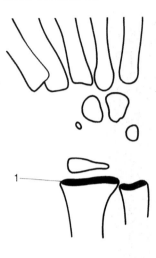

Observations

■ Dense line in the metaphysis involving distal radius and ulna due to deposition of lead (Atomic number = 92) and reactive change.

Diagnosis

LEAD POISONING: heavy metal deposition.

Notes

Ingestion of lead-containing paint (*pica*) was cause in this case. Diagnosis on plain abdominal X-ray showing dense flakes of paint in bowel. Confirmation by blood lead levels. Dense line seen most commonly at knees, wrists and ankles. Also occurs in other heavy metal poisoning (bismuth, mercury, phosphorus) and healed rickets.

CASE 15: Adult male

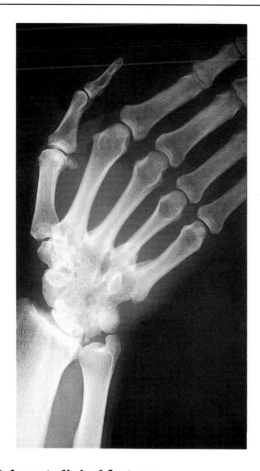

Relevant clinical features

■ Previous history of urethral discharge and inflamed left wrist.

■ Increasing stiffness and reduced movement of wrist.

CASE 15

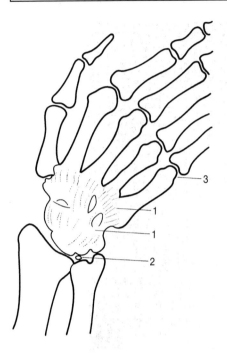

Observations
■ Fusion of carpal bones and carpometacarpal joints.
■ Loose body between radius and ulna.
■ MCP and other joints normal.

Diagnosis
BONY ANKYLOSIS: previous gonococcal infection.

Notes
Any chronic or inadequately treated infection (pyogenic or tuberculous) arthritis may cause bony ankylosis. Can also be due to severe non-infective arthropathies (rheumatoid or psoriatic) and is rarely the result of erosive osteoarthritis.

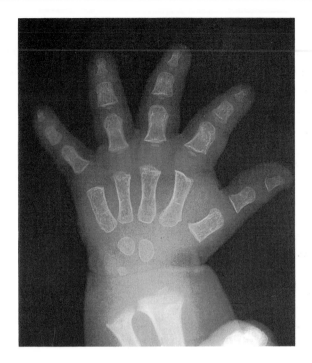

Relevant clinical features
- Dwarf.
- Enlarged head.
- Small face with sunken nasal bridge.

CASE 16

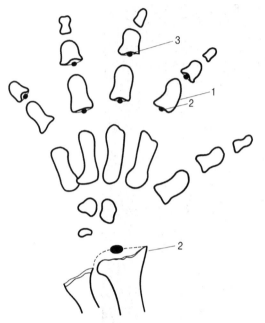

Observations
■ Tubular bones short wide and rectangular.
■ Metaphyseal cupping and irregularity.
■ All fingers of equal length and diverge from each other (trident hand).

Diagnosis
ACHONDROPLASIA: congenital bone dysplasia; retarded enchondral ossification.

Notes
Autosomal dominant inheritance. Commonest type of dwarfism. Short-limbed dwarfism affecting more the proximal bones of the limbs (rhizomelia). Many are stillborn or die in infancy from neurological complications.

■ Long bones and tubular bones: shortened with widened V-shaped metaphyses. Epiphyses very close to metaphyses.
■ Lumbar spine: interpedicular distance decreases from L1 to L5 due to tapering spinal canal. Leads to severe effects from spondylosis. Vertebral bodies flattened, scalloped posteriorly and some hypoplastic (wedge-shaped, *cf.* Hurler's syndrome (**Case 1** inset)).
■ Pelvis: small with squared ilia and horizontal acetabular roofs.
■ Skull: large cranium with short base, may be hydrocephalus.

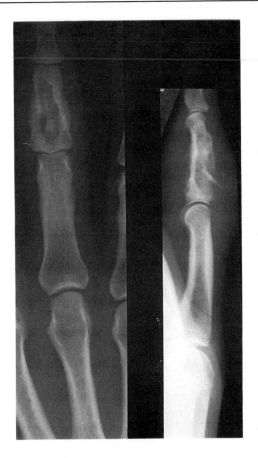

Relevant clinical features

■ Two-month history of painful swollen finger.

CASE 17

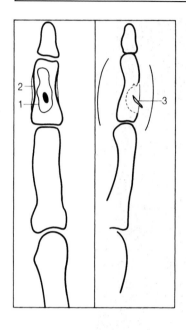

Observations

■ Extensive well-defined low-density area in the diaphysis of the middle phalanx (indicates medullary bone destruction as a result of infection).

■ The surrounding bone is widened and laminated due to periosteal new bone formation termed the involucrum.

■ Through dorsal defect in the involucrum (the cloaca) a dense spicule of dead bone (the sequestrum) is being extruded.

■ Other dead small bone fragments are seen in the swollen soft tissues.

Diagnosis

PYOGENIC OSTEOMYELITIS: haematogeneous bone infection.

Notes

Haematogeneous infection is usually to the metaphyses particularly in children. Predisposing factors include intravenous drug abuse, diabetes, sickle cell disease, immunosuppression, steroid therapy and white cell deficiency. Soft-tissue swelling after 3 days and radiographic changes (focus of reduced bone density) after 10 days. Spread of pus obliterates nutrient arteries and elevates periosteum, causing underlying bone death. Periosteum produces a shell of new bone – the involucrum. Through holes in these (cloacae) pus and dead bone fragments are discharged. Involucrum remodels with healing. With early treatment resolution of infection occurs without radiographic changes. With late or ineffective treatment tendency to chronicity. For osteomyelitis secondary to local soft tissue infection see *Case 13*.

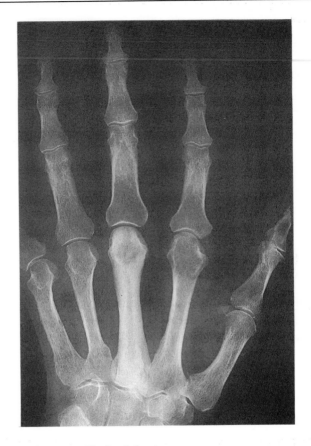

Relevant clinical features
■ Painful swelling on dorsum of hand, gradually developing over 6 months.

CASE 18

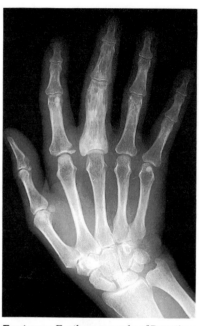

Observations
- Enlarged middle metacarpal.
- Cortex thickened.
- Trabecular pattern is coarse, arranged in a striated orientation and extends to the subarticular margin.
- Bone density increased (sclerotic).

Features: Further example of Paget's: expansion and thickened trabecular pattern affecting the proximal and middle phalanges of the middle finger.

Diagnosis
PAGET'S DISEASE: bone disease of unknown aetiology. Enlargement of the bone with increased bone density in an elderly skeleton.

Differential diagnosis
HAEMANGIOMA (coarse trabecular pattern) (see *Case 78*).

LYMPHOMAS (bone normal size) (see *Case 87*).

OSTEOBLASTIC METASTASES (bone normal size).

Notes
Condition commoner in males over age 60 years. Causes bone destruction and repair. Usually asymptomatic but may lead to deformities and fractures. Commonest in skull, lumbar spine, pelvis, femora and tibiae. In long and tubular bones always extends to the subarticular surface. Single or multiple bones involved. Softening of bone leads to deformities and fractures. Lytic variety in skull and tibia manifests as *osteoporosis circumscripta*. In the long bones, particularly the tibiae the lytic variety terminates in a 'V'. The sclerotic type gives enlargement of bones with coarse trabecular pattern or generalised increased bone density. Sarcomatous change in less than 1% of patients.

CASE 19: Adult male

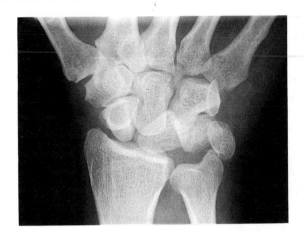

Relevant clinical features
- Fell off motorcycle.
- Injured both wrists.

CASE 19

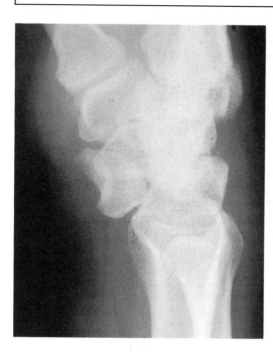

Observations

Posteroanterior view

- Lunate is triangular, i.e. has lost its normal trapezoidal shape.
- Carpus displaced proximally and in the ulnar direction.

Lateral view

- Volar (palmar) dislocation of lunate.
- Alignment of the distal radius to the distal carpal bones maintained (see inset).

Diagnosis

LUNATE DISLOCATION.

Notes

The scaphoid may also be dislocated with the lunate. If the scaphoid is fractured the proximal fragment is dislocated with the lunate.

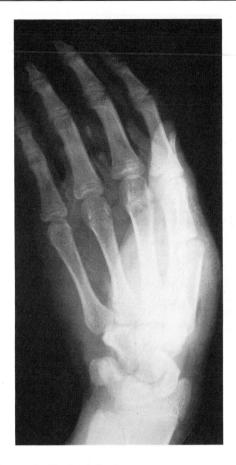

Relevant clinical features

■ Chest trauma.

CASE 20

Observations
■ Subcutaneous low-density linearities.

Diagnosis
SUBCUTANEOUS EMPHYSEMA: traumatic.

Notes
Due to escape of air into soft-tissue planes from breach of pleura, lung, trachea, bronchial tree, larynx or oesophagus. Chest, neck, face and arms involved in this case – 'Michelin man' appearance. Other causes include local open wounds and infection with gas forming organisms.

CASE 21: Male aged 30 years

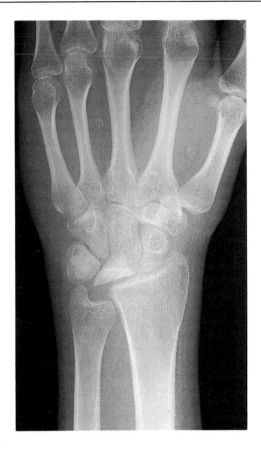

Relevant clinical features

■ Heavy manual worker.
■ Painful wrist, moderately swollen and tender.

CASE 21

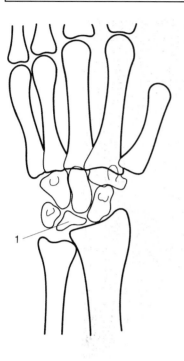

Observations

- Lunate irregular and partially collapsed with increased bone density (sclerotic).

Diagnosis

AVASCULAR NECROSIS OF THE LUNATE (syn. Kienbock's disease).

Notes

Single traumatic episode or recurrent trauma as in occupational cases, e.g. pneumatic-drill operators and woodworkers. Causes ischaemic death of the bone. Later (may be years) revascularisation, produces increased density. Liable to collapse or fragment. Subsequent degenerative change common.

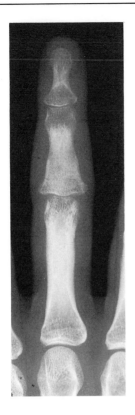

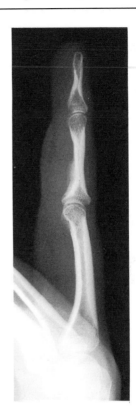

Relevant clinical features

■ One-month history of soft-tissue swelling of intermediate phalanx of middle finger with tenderness, limitation of movement and severe pain, worse at night.

■ Pain relieved by aspirin.

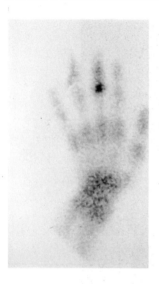

Observations
■ Base of intermediate phalanx widened.

■ Reactive new bone causing increased focal density.

■ Small ill-defined low-density 'nidus' is the osteoid osteoma.

■ Radionuclide bone scan shows focal uptake, base of middle phalanx.

Diagnosis
OSTEOID OSTEOMA: benign bone tumour.

Notes
Can occur at any site, but commonest in femur and tibia. Twice as common in males. Nidus can be medullary, intracortical, or subperiosteal and may calcify, i.e. appear dense. Nidus is not always visible on the plain films. High resolution CT using bone algorithm setting and axial 2–3 mm cuts may be required to identify the nidus. Differentiation must be made from chronic osteomyelitis, biopsy may be necessary. Treatment involves removing nidus.

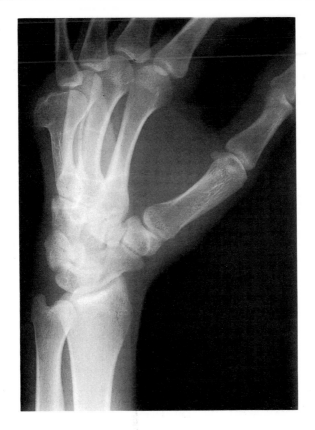

Relevant clinical features

■ Slowly growing hard lump.

CASE 23

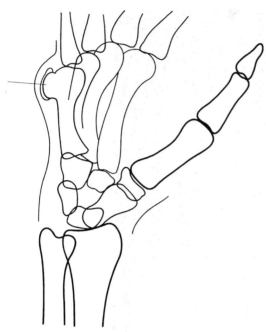

Observations
■ Broad-based bony mass on head of 5th metacarpal.

■ Mass has irregular cap and is directed away from the joint.

■ Cortex and bony trabeculae continuous with normal bone.

Diagnosis
SOLITARY OSTEOCHONDROMA (syn. cartilage capped exostosis): non-hereditary bone dysplasia.

Notes
Presents in second decade. Growth ceases with that of skeleton. Commonest around knee joint. Cartilage cap may calcify. Rarely becomes malignant.

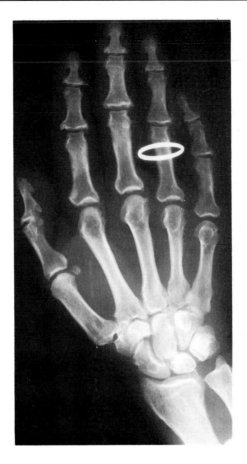

Relevant clinical features

■ Enlarged hands and feet.

■ Coarse facial features with large mandible.

CASE 24

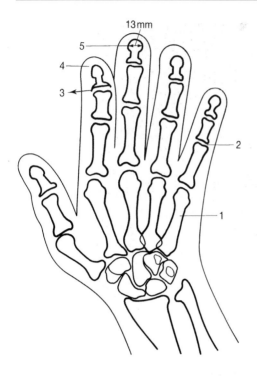

13mm
5
4
3
2
1

Observations
■ Metacarpals and phalanges, long and wide.
■ Articular spaces widened due to excess growth of cartilage and fibrous tissue.
■ Marginal spurs seen at the bases of the phalanges particularly the distal ones.
■ All soft tissues enlarged.
■ Terminal tufts 'spade-like' and enlarged: breadth >12 mm in male and >10 mm in female.

Diagnosis
ACROMEGALY: metabolic.

Notes
Excess pituitary growth hormone after epiphyseal closure leads to overgrowth of all tissues including soft tissue and cartilage. Visceromegaly also occurs. Typical facial appearance: large mandible, tongue, nose, thick lips, thickened coarse skin. Enlarged sella, sinuses and mastoids. Osteoarthritic changes seen in the hands and knees with subchondral cyst formation, bony outgrowth (spurs), but with preservation of normal or widened joint spaces. Osteoporosis and posterior scalloping of vertebral bodies may occur. Dysfunction of endocrine glands causes diabetes mellitus, hyperthyroidism and gonadal atrophy. Heel pad is thickened (>23 mm). Calcification of the pinna may occur.

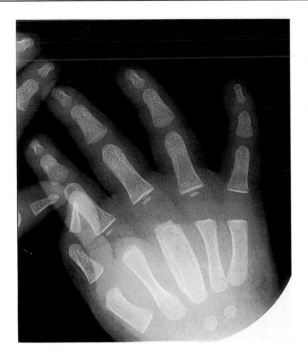

Relevant clinical features

■ Tender swelling of dorsum of right hand and outer border of left foot.

CASE 25

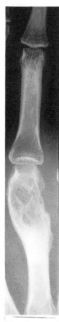

Observations
- Expanded 3rd metacarpal.
- Linear new bone formation (periosteal reaction) along the shaft.
- Soft-tissue swelling.

Features: *Spina ventosa: tuberculous dactylitis 3rd metacarpal in adult patient.*

Diagnosis
TUBERCULOUS DACTYLITIS: granulomatous osteomyelitis.

Notes
Common in ethnic minorities, particularly in children. Infection begins in metaphyses, spreads into shaft, crosses the growth plate into the epiphyses. Affected bone initially of low density then expands (spina ventosa). Cortex becomes destroyed. Associated with soft-tissue swelling, periosteal reaction, and areas of high density due to calcification.

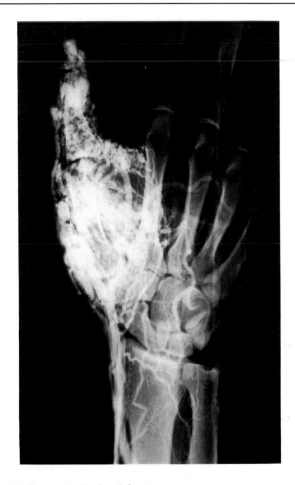

Relevant clinical features
- Knife wound to hand 2 years ago.
- Pulsatile swelling over thenar eminence.

CASE 26

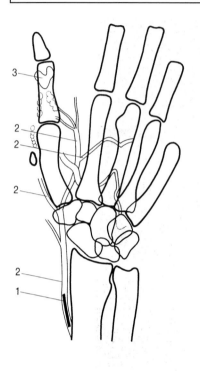

Observations
■ Selective angiogram of radial artery.

■ Very enlarged radial artery, princeps pollicis artery, digital arteries of the thumb, and arteries supplying the palmar arch.

■ Dilated veins over thumb and radial aspect of wrist which show early filling.

Diagnosis
POST-TRAUMATIC ARTERIOVENOUS FISTULA.

Notes
Almost all such fistulae are due to trauma (including iatrogenic). May cause pressure erosion of adjacent bone and if the shunt is large enough, can lead to cardiac failure.

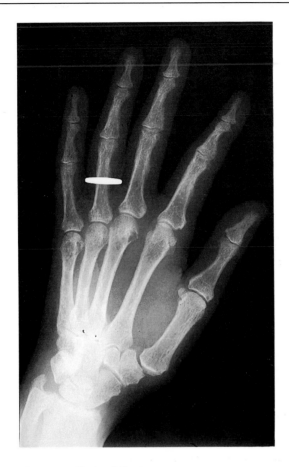

Relevant clinical features
- Bone pain, weakness, lethargy.
- Polydypsia, polyuria.

CASE 27

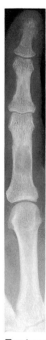

Features: *'Brown tumour' in proximal phalanx.*
Subperiosteal erosion in intermediate phalanx.
Tuft erosion of distal phalanx.

Observations

■ Generalised loss in bone density due to osteoporosis.

■ Sharp margin of cortical bone lost; best seen radial aspect middle and distal phalanges, i.e. 'subperiosteal bone resorption'.

■ Sparse coarse trabecular pattern.

■ Rounded low-density (cyst-like lesion) head of meta carpal of middle finger, i.e. 'brown tumour'.

Diagnosis

PRIMARY HYPERPARATHYROIDISM: metabolic.

Differential diagnosis

SECONDARY HYPERPARATHYROIDISM: bones similar but may be more dense and brown tumours uncommon. Serum calcium usually low.

Notes

Due to parathyroid adenoma, hyperplasia or carcinoma or non-parathyroid tumours secreting parathormone-like substances. Resulting increase in osteoclastic bone resorption with raised serum calcium and alkaline phosphatase. Earliest radiographic change is subperiosteal bone resorption. Other bone eroded include clavicle, ribs, tibia, symphysis pubis, sacroiliac joints, skull ('pepper pot') and lamina dura. Softening of bone causes deformities and fractures. *Brown tumours* in 3%. Hypercalcaemia leads to renal calculi, nephrocalcinosis and metastatic calcification.

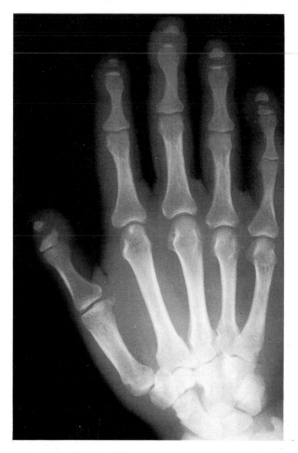

Relevant clinical features

- Tenderness of fingertips.
- Raynaud's phenomenon, both hands.
- Skin nodules on dorsum of hands and forearm.

CASE 28

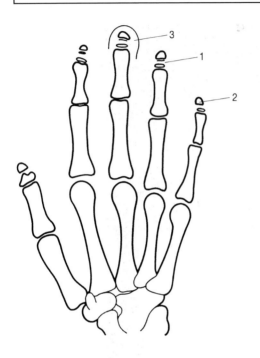

Observations
■ Absent bone in centres of terminal phalanges – 'slice defects'.

■ Several terminal phalangeal tufts irregular with half-moon appearance.

■ Clubbing of fingers.

Diagnosis
VINYL CHLORIDE POISONING: occupational acro-osteolysis.

Notes
May progress to complete resorption of tufts. After removal from toxic exposure, fibrous and bony union occurs. Associated sacroiliitis and liver haemangiosarcoma have been described. Causes of acro-osteolysis are:

■ Collagen diseases: scleroderma, dermatomyositis, Ehlers–Danlos syndrome, Raynaud's disease.
■ Injuries: frostbite, burns, electric shock.
■ Arthropathies: rheumatoid, Reiter's syndrome, psoriasis.
■ Granulomatous infection: leprosy, sarcoidosis.
■ Endocrine: hyperparathyroidism primary and secondary.

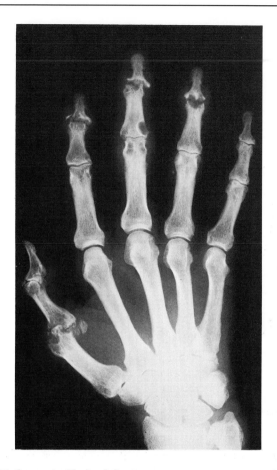

Relevant clinical features

■ Red scaly patches around elbows and knees.

■ Painful joint swellings of fingers and thumb of both hands, particularly the distal joints of the fingers.

■ Pitted nails.

CASE 29

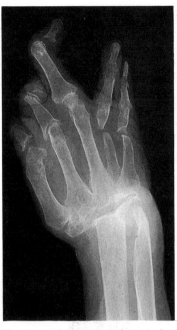

Observations

■ Sharply marginated areas of extensive destruction ('erosions') in articular surfaces of DIP joints of index, middle, ring fingers, PIP joint of middle finger and MCP joint of thumb.

■ Cupping of bases of distal phalanges with widening of the joint spaces in the affected areas.

Features: Arthritis mutilans: indistinguishable from rheumatoid. DIP joints subluxed.

Diagnosis

PSORIATIC ARTHRITIS: seronegative arthropathy.

Differential diagnosis

EROSIVE ARTHROPATHIES: rheumatoid arthritis (see **Case 3**), reticulohistiocytoma (lipoddermatoarthritis).

Notes

Asymmetrical peripheral erosive arthritis in over 10% of all psoriasis patients, most commonly when rash on palms and soles and nails affected. Rarely joint involvement precedes the rash. In patients with psoriasis and arthritis one-third have classical psoriatic arthritis, one-third have rheumatoid-type arthritis and one-third have features of both (see inset). Radiographic changes:

■ Erosions: in DIP joints – may lead to cup and pencil deformity.
■ Joint spaces: widened.
■ Periosteal reactions: mainly in phalanges and hallux metatarsal.
■ Lack of osteoporosis.

■ Distribution: more common in hands than in feet. Spinal involvement may give atlantoaxial subluxation, spondylitis and sacroiliitis.
■ Complications: arthritis mutilans, (see inset), bony ankylosis.

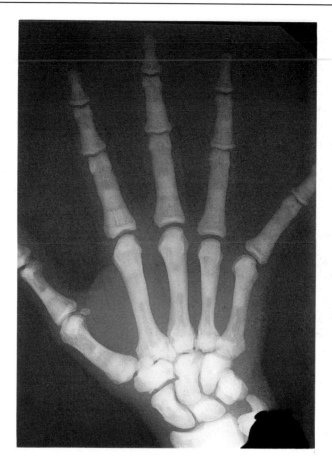

Relevant clinical features
- Anaemia.
- Bleeding gums.

CASE 30

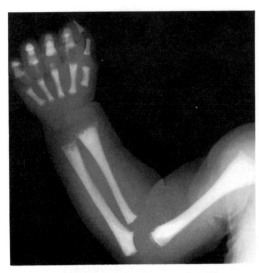

Observations

■ Uniform symmetrical increase in bone density (sclerosis).

■ Distinction between cortex and medulla tends to be lost with narrowing of medullary cavities.

■ Miniature inset of bone seen in the metacarpals and phalanges giving the 'bone-within-a-bone appearance'.

■ Multiple low density transverse striations.

Features: Neonatal type with generalised bone sclerosis.

Diagnosis

OSTEOPETROSIS: (Marble bone disease; Albers–Schonberg disease) hereditary bone dysplasia.

Notes

Bone resorption and formation impaired with persisting calcified cartilage leads to dense brittle bones. Bones may be totally sclerotic or partially sclerotic producing transverse low-density bands or 'bone-within-a-bone' appearance. Two types: *autosomal recessive* (see inset) clinically malignant. Stillbirth or neonatal death or presents before age of 10 years. Bones are brittle and fracture with minimal trauma. Loss of medullary cavities leads to anaemia, thrombocytopenia, hepatosplenomegaly. Foraminal narrowing in skull causes optic atrophy and facial nerve palsy. *Autosomal dominant* (tarda form): relatively benign. Presents in adult usually with a fracture. Bones patchily sclerotic. May be a thick skull vault, dense bands in vertebral bodies. Dentition is defective leading to osteomyelitis of mandible and maxilla. Increased mortality due to haemorrhage, infection or leukaemia.

CASE 31: Adult male

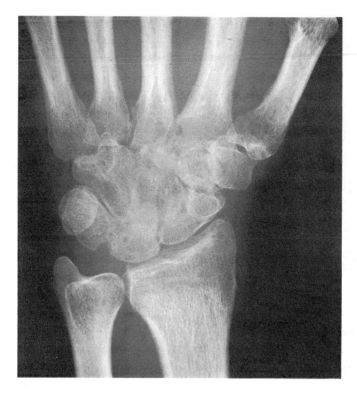

Relevant clinical features

■ Increasing pain and swelling of wrist for 2 weeks.

■ Fever.

CASE 31

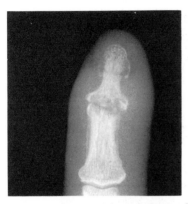

Features: *Acute pyogenic arthritis of distal interphalangeal joint following puncture wound. Periosteal reaction along intermediate phalanx from spread of infection along bone.*

Observations

■ Generalised loss in bone density affecting carpal bones: osteoporosis (due to hyperaemia).

■ Narrowing of the joint spaces (due to cartilage destruction).

■ Loss of definition of carpal bones, particularly the capitate (due to erosion of subchondral bone).

Diagnosis

PYOGENIC ARTHRITIS: infective arthropathy.

Differential diagnosis

TUBERCULOUS ARTHRITIS (see **Case 37**).

RHEUMATOID ARTHRITIS (see **Case 19**).

REFLEX SYMPATHETIC DYSTROPY SYNDROME (see **Case 11**).

Notes

Usually haematogeneous infection with staphylococci, streptococci or pneumococci. These produce proteolytic enzymes which cause early cartilage and subchondral bone destruction. May lead to subluxation and ankylosis. Appropriate early antibiotic therapy would be expected to prevent destructive lesions.

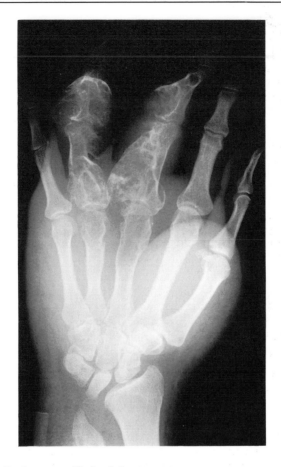

Relevant clinical features

■ Hard painful swelling of middle and ring fingers.

■ Shortened and bowed forearm.

CASE 32

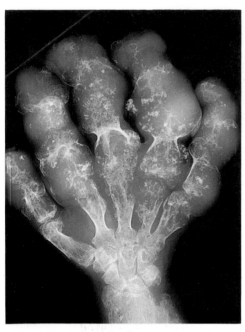

Features: *Gross example of multiple enchondromatosis. Note high density foci of calcification.*

Observations

■ Markedly expanded proximal and intermediate phalanges of middle and ring fingers.

■ Protrusions, due to multiple well-defined low-density lesions at the bases of these phalanges.

■ Less marked changes in associated metacarpal heads.

■ Associated Madelung's deformity (see **Case 50**).

Diagnosis

MULTIPLE ENCHONDROMATOSIS: (syn. Ollier's disease) non-hereditary osseous dysplasia.

Notes

Due to hypertrophy of cartilage at growth plates. No further enlargement in mature skeleton. Can involve any bone. Articular surfaces remain intact. Unilateral form termed Ollier's disease. Sarcomatous change is common, especially in Maffucci's syndrome. (Soft-tissue haemangiomas associated with enchondromatoses.)

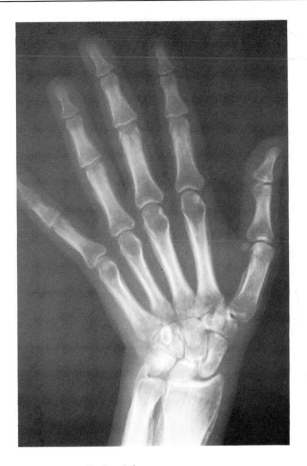

Relevant clinical features

■ Clubbing of fingers.

■ Painful wrists.

■ Erythematous rim surrounding base of nails.

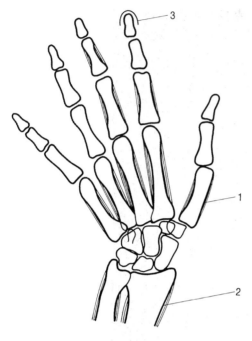

Observations

■ Irregular linear density along cortex of diaphyses of all tubular bones, metacarpals and phalanges, i.e. new bone from periosteal reaction.

■ Distal radius and ulna also involved.

■ Soft-tissue swelling over tufts (clubbing).

■ Symmetrical changes in both hands and wrists.

Diagnosis

HYPERTROPHIC OSTEOARTHROPATHY: primary periosteal/joint/soft-tissue disease.

Differential diagnosis

THYROID ACROPACHY: vertical feathery periosteal reaction metacarpals and phalanges does not involve radius and ulna. (See **Case 12**.)

PACHYDERMOPERIOSTOSIS: non-tender periostitis; hyperhydrosis of hands and feet. (See **Case 36**.)

Notes

Triad composed of periosteal new bone formation, clubbing (i.e. soft-tissue swelling over tufts but no bony abnormality of distal phalanges) and synovitis. Periostitis may affect long bones around elbows, knees, ankles and feet. This case associated with primary bronchial carcinoma. Radiographic changes in such cases regress slowly after vagotomy, resection or radiotherapy. Causes of HOA:

■ Chronic lung infection: abscess, bronchiectasis, cystic fibrosis, tuberculosis.
■ Tumours of the lung: adenoma, carcinoma, mesothelioma, metastasis.
■ Heart disease: cyanotic congenital.
■ Bowel and liver disease: cirrhosis, ulcerative colitis and Crohn's disease.

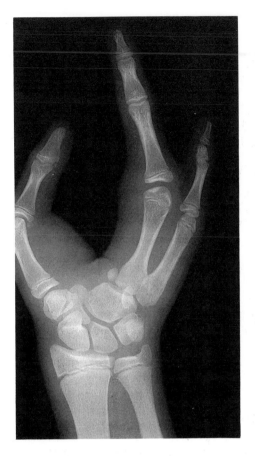

Relevant clinical features

■ Deformity of one hand.

■ Hare lip and cleft palate.

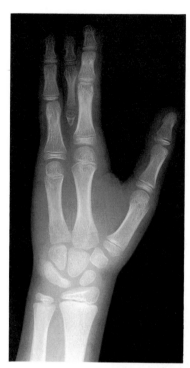

Observations

■ Index and middle fingers and their metacarpals absent.

■ Small middle phalanx of little finger.

■ Enlarged bone and soft tissue of ring finger.

Features: Another example. Additional hypoplastic phalanges between index and middle fingers.

Diagnosis

LOBSTER CLAW (SPLIT-HAND) DEFORMITY: congenital abnormality.

Notes

Many variations on this central hypoplasia. Genetically related to other types of hypoplasia of hand including monodactyly. May be unilateral or bilateral. Associated abnormalities include cleft palate and lip, cleft foot, mandibulofacial dysostosis, cataracts, congenital nystagmus, anonychia, cyclopia, congenital heart disease and imperforate anus.

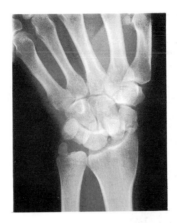

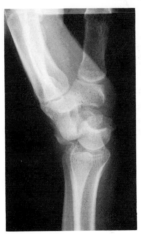

Relevant clinical features

- Road traffic accident.
- Swelling and tenderness of wrist.

CASE 35

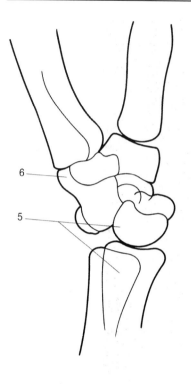

Observations

Frontal view

■ Transverse irregular low density line horizontally through the waist of the scaphoid with separation of the fragments.

■ Triangular appearance to the lunate.

■ Distal row of carpal bones misaligned with proximal row.

■ Low-density line in ulnar styloid.

Lateral view

■ Lunate aligned with radius; proximal fragments of scaphoid remains with lunate.

■ Capitate displaced dorsally.

Diagnosis

TRANSCAPHOID PERILUNATE FRACTURE DISLOCATION OF WRIST: fracture of ulnar styloid and triquetrum.

Notes

Rarely the dislocation may be in a volar (palmar) direction. Note: the lunate remains aligned to the radius, the distal row of carpal bones are displaced in either a dorsal or volar direction.

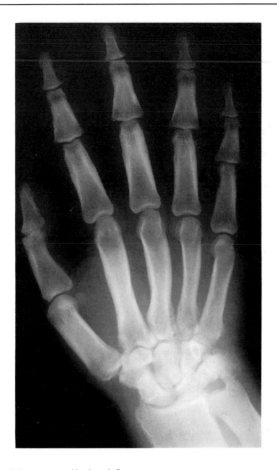

Relevant clinical features

■ Increasing thickening of the skin affecting the face, hands, forearms, feet and lower legs.

■ Long-standing finger clubbing.

■ Non-tender distal extremities.

CASE 36

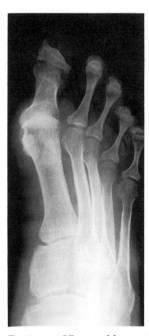

Features: *37 year old man with soft tissue swelling and resorption of the distal phalanx first toe.*

Observations

■ Cortical thickening along all metacarpal shafts, proximal and middle phalanges.
■ Marked soft-tissue swelling.

Diagnosis

PACHYDERMOPERIOSTOSIS: primary benign inherited thickening of bone and soft tissue.

Differential diagnosis

THYROID ACROPACHY: (see *Case 12*).

HYPERTROPHIC PULMONARY OSTEOARTHROPATHY: (see *Case 33*).

ACROMEGALY: (see *Case 24*).

Notes

Autosomal dominant familial condition. More common in males. Usually begins at puberty progressing for several years then ceasing. Cortical thickening involves distal ends of long bones, hands and feet which are widened, and periosteal new bone merges with the cortex and narrows the medullary canal. Distal phalanges rarely involved but may be associated with gross acro-osteolysis (see inset). Soft-tissue thickening involves the face. There is associated with clubbing of the fingers and enlarged sinuses.

CASE 37: Indian adult male

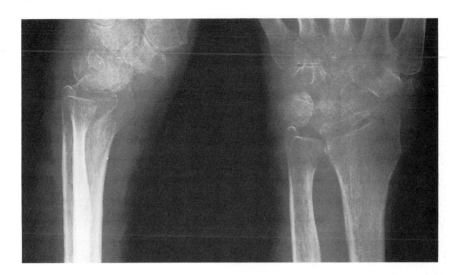

Relevant clinical features
- Gradual onset over several months of swelling and moderate pain in left wrist.
- Other joints normal.

CASE 37

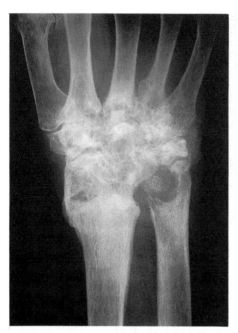

Observations
■ Low density of bones with hazy outlines (osteoporosis due to hyperaemia).
■ Soft-tissue swelling.

Features: More advanced case showing erosions of carpal and ulnar carpal joint. Erosions with associated ankylosis of radiocarpal joint.

Diagnosis
TUBERCULOUS ARTHRITIS: infective arthropathy.

Differential diagnosis
PYOGENIC ARTHRITIS: acute onset and early destruction of articular surfaces (see *Case 31*).

RHEUMATOID ARTHRITIS: usually involves more than one joint (see *Cases 3* and *92*).

Notes
Tuberculosis arthritis usually monoarticular. Occurs in 10% of pulmonary tuberculosis cases. Commonest in spine (50%) and hip (30%). Insidious onset. Initially synovitis with osteoporosis and joint effusion. Only later (due to lack of proteolytic enzymes) is the articular cartilage and then the subarticular bone destroyed. Healing causes increased bone density, soft-tissue calcification, and possibly ankylosis (see inset).

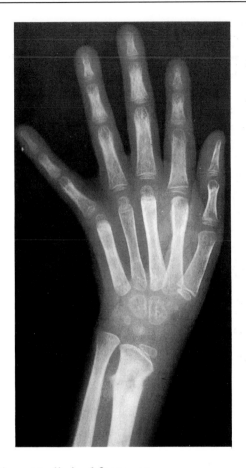

Relevant clinical features

■ Painful swollen hands and feet.

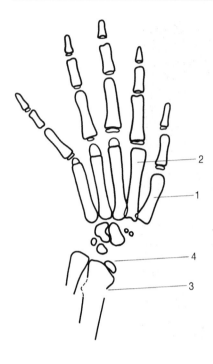

Observations
■ Low-density widened medullary cavities (thumb metacarpal) due to marrow hyperplasia.

■ Other bones show patchy increase in bone density due to infarcts.

■ Distal radius fragmented due to infarction/infection.

■ Radiocarpal subluxation.

Diagnosis
SICKLE CELL DISEASE (Hb SS): haemoglobinopathy.

Notes
Combination of medullary hyperplasia and infarction in a black child is typical of this disease. Infection resulting from *Salmonella paratyphi* B in endemic areas.

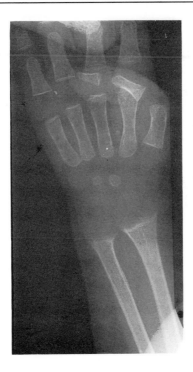

Relevant clinical features

■ Born prematurely.

■ Swollen joints and costochondral junctions.

CASE 39

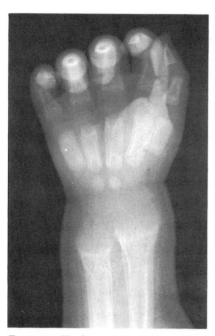

Observations
■ Metaphyseal margins look frayed and ill defined (due to poorly calcified bone).
■ Metaphyseal cupping and widening (due to weakening).
■ Generalised reduction in bone density (osteoporosis).

Features: Healing rickets: two months following treatment, periosteal reaction along the diaphyses and increased density of distal radius and ulnar metaphyses.

Diagnosis
RICKETS: vitamin D deficiency bone disease.

Notes
Softening of bone may lead to fractures and bowing of bones. Delayed ossification. May be due to dietary calcium deficiency, deficiency of or resistance to vitamin D, malabsorptive states, liver disease, renal disease, or anticonvulsant medication.

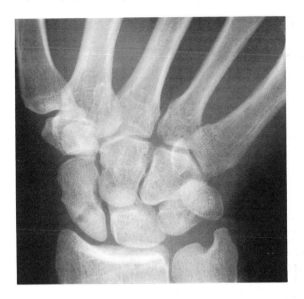

Relevant clinical features
- Pain in wrist.
- Fell on outstretched hand 18 months ago.
- Did not attend for treatment.

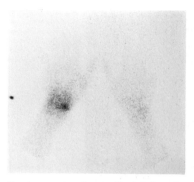

Observations

■ Low-density line through proximal pole of scaphoid (indicating old ununited fracture).

■ Increased density (sclerosis) proximal pole fragment of scaphoid (due to revascularisation of necrotic bone).

Features: *Another patient: Injury 6 months previously; immobilised in scaphoid plaster. Radiograph normal. Patient remains symptomatic. Bone scan: increased uptake of radioactive isotope (^{99m}Tc MDP) in region of scaphoid.*

Diagnosis

OSTEONECROSIS: proximal pole of scaphoid.

Notes

A branch of the radial artery enters the waist of the scaphoid and supplies all the bone except for the distal pole. Fractures of the waist and, in particular, the proximal pole if not adequately treated (immobilised early) result in ischaemic necrosis with delayed union or non-union. This may be as high as 30–50% in fractures of the proximal pole. Further imaging options include radionuclide bone scan, computerised tomography (CT), or magnetic resonance imaging (MRI) scans. These additional investigations are particularly useful in patients with occult fractures (plain X-rays normal) and who remain symptomatic.

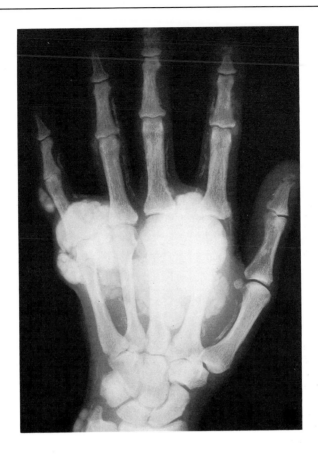

Relevant clinical features
■ Chronic renal failure on dialysis.
■ Hard painless swellings on hands.

CASE 41

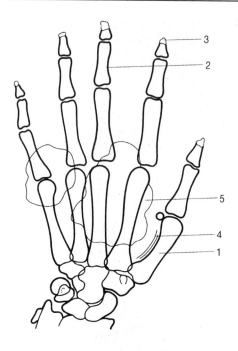

Observations

- Generalised increased density of bones (osteosclerosis).
- Irregular scalloping of radial aspects of intermediate phalanges (subperiosteal resorption).
- Partial destruction of terminal phalanges.
- Arterial calcification.
- Large calcified deposits in soft tissues.

Diagnosis

RENAL OSTEODYSTROPHY: metabolic bone disease.

Notes

In the adult chronic renal failure produces a low serum calcium which causes osteomalacia evident as low bone density associated with Looser's zones (i.e. pseudofractures typically in ribs, scapulae and femoral necks). In some cases the high serum phosphate/calcium ratio results in vascular and soft tissue calcification. Secondary hyperparathyroidism induces increased osteoclastic activity which may produce subperiosteal and tuft erosions. Osteosclerosis may occur (as in this case); its cause is unknown.

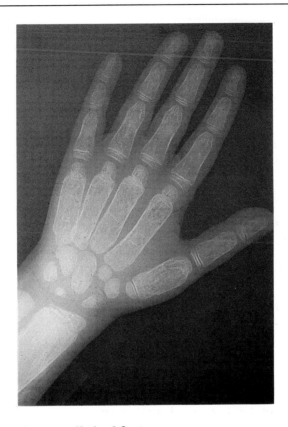

Relevant clinical features
- Severe anaemia.
- Jaundice.
- Hepatosplenomegaly.
- Bossing of skull.

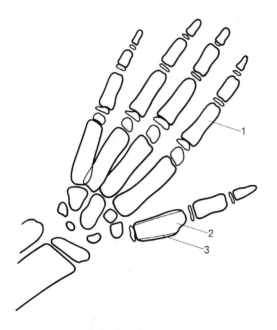

Observations
■ Generalised loss in bone density (osteoporosis).
■ Medullary spaces expanded (metacarpals biconvex) due to marrow hyperplasia.
■ Cortices thinned.

Diagnosis
THALASSEMIA MAJOR: haemoglobinopathy.

Differential diagnosis
CONGENITAL SKELETAL ANOMALIES/DYSPLASIA: (i.e. mucopolysaccharidoses, Gaucher's and Engelmann's disease) have expanded bones of low density. For differentiating features see **Cases 1, 88** and **6**, respectively.

Notes
Homozygous form presents in infancy. Causes gross hyperplasia of the marrow affecting majority of the skeleton. In skull diploic spaces widened assuming 'hair-on-end' appearance. Large paraspinal soft tissue masses due to extramedullary haemopoiesis. Premature fusion of epiphyses leads to stunted growth. Apart from expansion, no deformity is present.

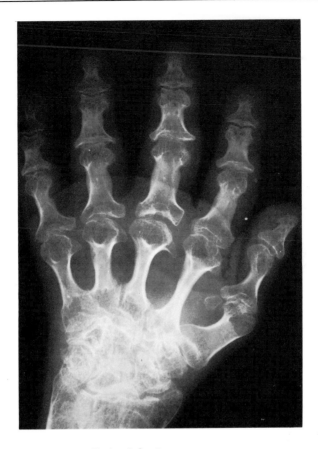

Relevant clinical features

■ Short-limbed dwarf.

■ Small hands with short stubby fingers.

CASE 43

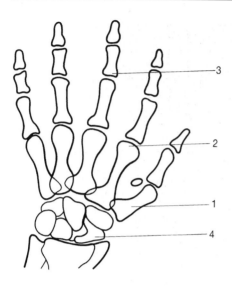

Observations
- All tubular bones short.
- Broad irregular epiphyses.
- Splaying of several metaphyses.
- Carpal bones misshapen and small.

Diagnosis
PSEUDOACHONDROPLASTIC DYSPLASIA.

Notes
Autosomal dominant inheritance. This form of short-limb dwarfism resembles achondroplasia clinically but is not evident at birth. Spinal involvement is a prominent feature of this condition, causing flattening of vertebral bodies with a localised kyphosis. Involvement of hips leads to early degenerative changes. Face and skull not involved.

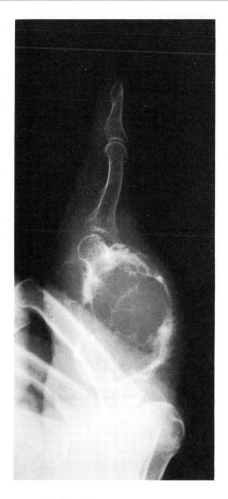

Relevant clinical features
- Hard swelling of middle finger.
- Enlarging over 2 years.
- Recently painful.

CASE 44

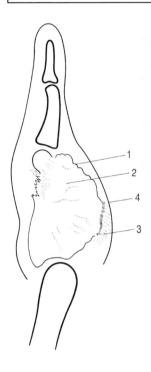

Observations
■ Whole proximal phalanx expanded (solitary lesion) with scalloped endosteal margins.

■ Multiple low-density ill-defined areas.

■ Bony spicules from outer layer of cortex penetrating into the soft tissues.

■ Soft-tissue swelling.

Diagnosis
CHONDROSARCOMA: primary malignant cartilage tumour.

Notes
Solitary bone lesion associated with above aggressive radiological features suggests primary bone malignancy. Chondrosarcomas are common over 40 years of age. Slow growing, but eventually metastasises to lung. Commonest in the femur. Most show calcification. Sarcomatous changes may occur in osteochondroma, diaphyseal aclasia, enchondromatosis and Paget's disease. Malignant features include pain, soft-tissue swelling, rapid growth, wide zone of transition between normal and abnormal bone, cortical spiculation and/or bone destruction.

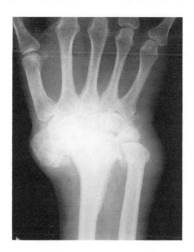

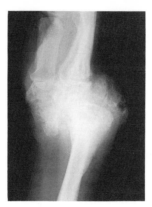

Relevant clinical features
■ Painless deformed wrist.
■ Hard swelling around wrist.

CASE 45

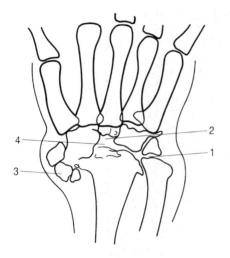

Observations
- Dislocation of radiocarpal joint.
- Increased bone density.
- Multiple osseous particles around joint.
- Deformed articular surfaces with narrowed joint spaces.
- Resulting disorganisation of carpus.

Diagnosis
NEUROPATHIC ARTHROPATHY: (syn. Charcot's joint) hypertrophic form.

Notes
Repeated trauma in absence of pain leads to gross degenerative changes. The atrophic type shows osteoporosis, resorption of bone ends and joint effusion. Causes include:

- CNS and spinal lesions: neurosyphilis, syringomyelia, spinabifida, meningomyelocele.
- Peripheral neuropathy: diabetes, leprosy, congenital absence of pain.
- Joint therapy: intra-articular steroid injections.

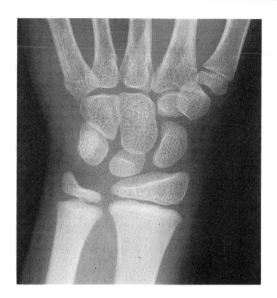

Relevant clinical features

■ Hirsute and muscular.

CASE 46

Observations

■ Skeletal maturity at 9 years.[*]

Diagnosis

ADVANCED SKELETAL MATURATION: due to adrenogenital syndrome.

Notes

Autosomal recessive inheritance. Clinically evident in the homozygous state. Commoner in females. Enzyme deficiency (usually C-21 hydroxylase) results in impaired cortisol production and increased ACTH secretion. This leads to adrenal hyperplasia and excessive androgen metabolites. Causes virilisation in girls and precocious puberty in boys. Other causes of advanced skeletal maturation include tumours of pituitary, parapituitary area, adrenal liver and gonads, hyperthyroidism and various congenital abnormalities (e.g. fibrous dysplasia, Beckwith–Wiedemann syndrome). Mild advancement in skeletal maturation is common in obesity and may be idiopathic.

[*] W. W. Greulich and S. I. Pyle, *Radiographic Atlas of Skeletal Development of the Hand and Wrist*, Stanford University Press, Stanford, CA.

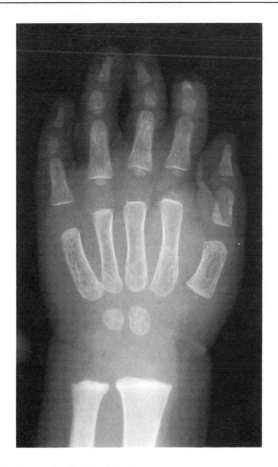

Relevant clinical features
■ Fusion of web spaces between index/middle and middle/ring fingers.
■ Absence of sternocostal portion of right pectoralis major muscle and right nipple.

CASE 47

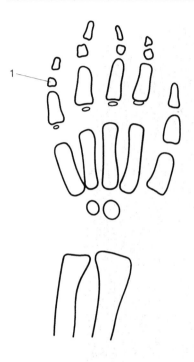

1

Observations
■ Short intermediate pha-lanx of all fingers.

Diagnosis
POLAND'S SYNDROME: (syn. pectoral aplasia – dysdactyly syndrome).

Notes
Sporadic condition with characteristic abnormalities, usually in males. Unilateral, commonly right-sided. Infant otherwise normal. Unknown cause: may be due to hypoplasia of the subclavian artery.

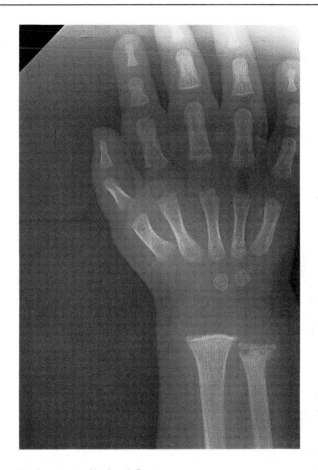

Relevant clinical features
- Tender swollen joints.
- Extensive bruising.

CASE 48

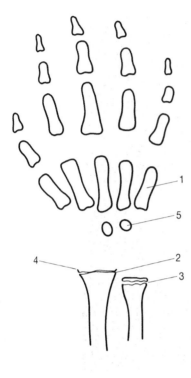

Observations

■ Reduced density of bones with thin cortices: indicates osteoporosis.

■ Metaphyseal dense band: due to persisting calcification of cartilage.

■ Subjacent low-density band (Truemmerfeld zone): due to deficient ossification.

■ Metaphyseal marginal spurs (Pelkan spurs): healing of associated fractures.

■ Cortex of epiphyses relatively dense: ring appearance (Wimbergers sign).

Diagnosis

SCURVY: vitamin C deficiency disease.

Notes

Rare under 6 months. Spontaneous fractures may occur at weakened metaphyses. Subperiosteal bleeding leads to extensive new bone formation. Rapid healing following introduction of mixed diet and treatment with vitamin C.

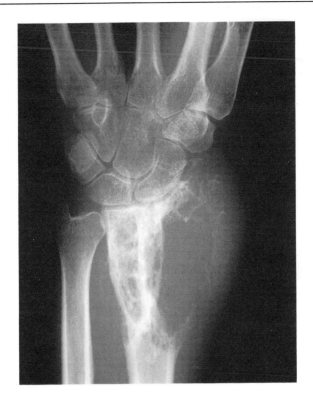

Relevant clinical features
■ Increasing swelling of left wrist.
■ Associated intermittent dull ache for 6 months.

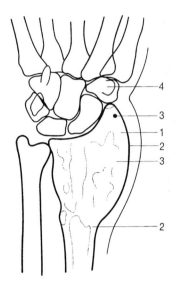

Observations

■ Large expansile low-density (destructive) lesion in distal radius off central axis and extending to the articular surface.

■ The transition zone between pathological and normal bone not clear-cut, indicating that the lesion is not benign.

■ Some trabecula preserved.

■ Carpal bones: diffuse loss of bone density.

Diagnosis

GIANT CELL TUMOUR: primary bone tumour.

Differential diagnosis

EXPANDING SOLITARY LESION IN YOUNG ADULT.

ANEURYSMAL BONE CYST: expansile well-defined cyst which extends to epiphyseal plate. 75% of patients are young, i.e. before epiphyseal closure.

BROWN TUMOURS OF HYPERPARATHYROIDISM: (check blood calcium) (see **Case 27**).

FIBROUS DYSPLASIA: (see **Case 58**).

CHONDROBLASTOMA: arises after epiphyseal closure – extends from articular margin into metaphyses; varying amounts of spotty calcification may be present.

Notes

Almost always solitary. Radiological appearances variable with grade of malignancy, i.e. margins of more malignant tumours are poorly defined. Usually 20–40 years old. Rarely in association with Paget's disease. May recur, or metastasise after excision, embolisation or radiotherapy.

CASE 50: Female aged 18 years

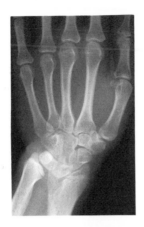

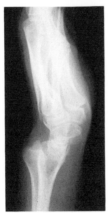

Relevant clinical features

■ Deformities at both wrists.

■ Short stature.

CASE 50

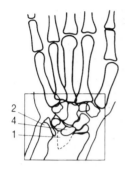

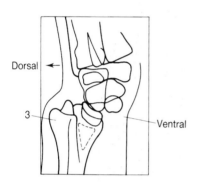

Dorsal ←

3

Ventral

Observations
■ V-shaped low density of medial aspect of distal radial epiphysis and metaphysis (due to premature fusion leading to asymmetrical growth).
■ Ulna head is abnormally shaped.
■ Dorsal subluxation of ulna on lateral film.
■ Carpal bones become wedged between the deformity with lunate at apex.

Diagnosis
MADELUNG'S DEFORMITY: congenital cartilage dysplasia.

Notes
Usually bilateral. Commoner in females. May be part of a generalised bone dysplasia – this patient is a dyschondrosteosis dwarf with short lower limbs. Madelung's deformity can be associated with enchondromatosis, multiple exostoses, Turner's syndrome. Unilateral lesions more likely to develop as a result of previous trauma.

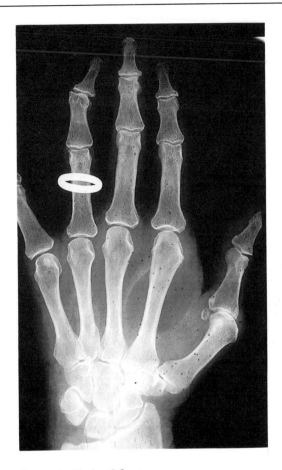

Relevant clinical features
■ Painless soft-tissue swelling in palm.
■ Present for several years.

CASE 51

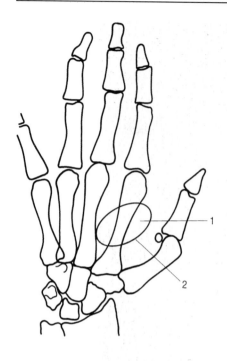

Observations
- Low-density (fat density) 4 cm mass over index meta-carpal.
- Smooth sharply demarcated margins.

(Black dots are artifactual)

Diagnosis
LIPOMA OF SOFT TISSUES: benign fat–containing neoplasm.

Notes
Common, especially in middle-aged females. May be multiple. Rarely calcifies and may cause pressure effects on nerves and bones.

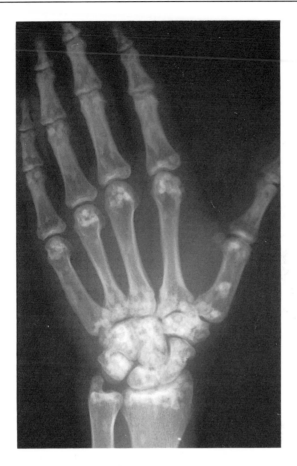

Relevant clinical features

■ Incidental findings in patient examined following trauma.

CASE 52

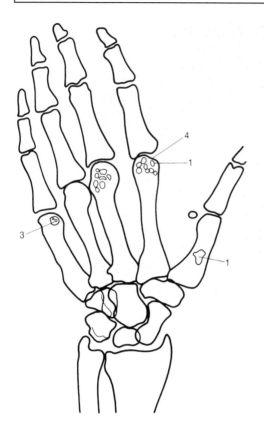

Observations
■ Small rounded foci of increased density.
■ Few millimetres to a few centimetres in size.
■ Low-density centres.
■ Nearer the ends of bones, i.e. in epiphyses and metaphyses.

Diagnosis
OSTEOPOIKILOSIS: hereditary bone disorder.

Notes
Autosomal dominant inheritance. Does not progress. No clinical significance. May be associated with other conditions including dermatofibrosis, scleroderma, syndactyly, dwarfism, melorheostosis, endocrine abnormalities and cleft palate.

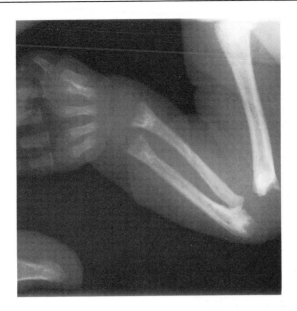

Relevant clinical features
- Failure to thrive.
- Bowed legs.

CASE 53

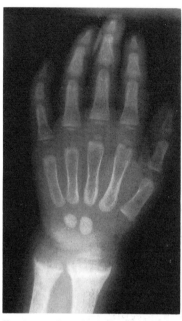

Observations
- Metaphyses irregular.
- Generalised loss in bone density (osteopenia).
- Characteristic sharp deep defects seen at the wrist joint and around elbow joint.
- Slight bowing of the long bones.

Features: Renal tubular hypophosphataemic rickets due to impaired resorption of phosphate from proximal tubules. Low serum phosphate. Note the increased bone density as well as changes of rickets.

Diagnosis
INFANTILE HYPOPHOSPHATAEMIA.

Differential diagnosis
RICKETS: from other causes. (See inset and *Case 39*.)

Notes
Hypophosphataemia is a metaphyseal dysplasia with reduction in the activity of alkaline phosphatase leading to incomplete ossification of cartilage and increased urinary phosphorylethanolamine. Serum phosphate normal. Radiological changes seen are similar to those in dietary rickets, but the sharp deep metaphyseal defects are characteristic. Radiological appearance correlates into four age groups:

- Congenital neonatal hypophosphataemia: results in little bone mineralisation and often causes stillbirth; may resemble osteogenesis imperfecta.
- Infantile hypophosphataemia: changes less severe. Soft-tissue calcification due to hypercalcemia.
- Childhood hypophosphataemia: defective gait, short stature, painful extremities.
- Adult hypophosphataemia: mild form with bowing of long bones and pseudofractures.

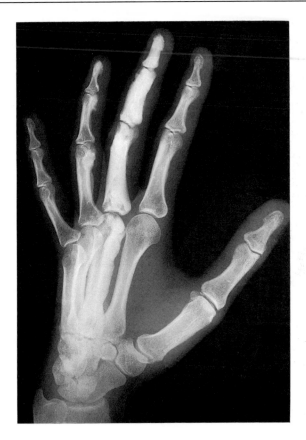

Relevant clinical features
■ Pains and stiffness in the middle and ring fingers of the hand.
■ Symptoms since childhood.

CASE 54

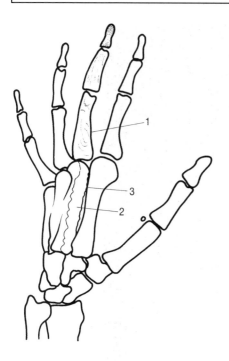

Observations
■ Thickened cortex due to periosteal and endosteal new bone formation.
■ One side of bone more involved.
■ Affected bones enlarged.
■ Hyperostosis likened to wax dripping along the side of a burning candle.

Diagnosis
MELORHEOSTOSIS: bone dysplasia.

Notes
Increased bone can interfere with joint movement, compress nerves and blood vessels. Condition segmental and usually unilateral. Sometimes bilateral but asymmetrical. May be scleroderma-like changes in skin.

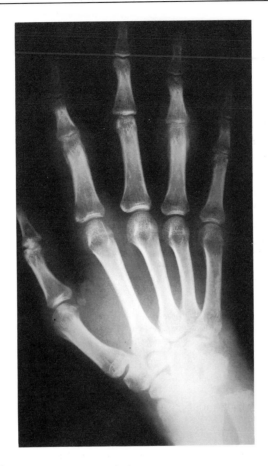

Relevant clinical features

■ Soft-tissue swelling of over the PIP joints of index and ring finger.

■ Urethritis.

■ Conjunctivitis.

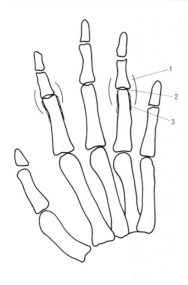

Observations

- Soft-tissue swelling of over the PIP joints of index and ring fingers.
- Narrowing of affected joint spaces.
- Linear new bone along the proximal phalanges (periosteal reaction).

Diagnosis

REITER'S SYNDROME: inflammatory arthropathy.

Differential diagnosis

Other inflammatory arthropathies including:

RHEUMATOID ARTHRITIS.

PSORIATIC ARTHROPATHY.

ANKLOSING SPONDYLYTIS.

Notes

Triad of arthritis, conjunctivitis and urethritis. Almost entirely confined to males and usually a sexually transmitted disease but a similar syndrome without urethritis may follow dysentery. Characteristic skin rash keratodermia blennorrhagium. Asymmetrical arthritis involving most commonly the sacroiliac joints, MTP and tarsal joints and, less commonly, the hips and knees and usually the wrists and hands. Plantar fasciitis with calcaneum spurs common. Like rheumatoid arthritis, but male preponderance, asymmetrical, exuberant periosteal new bone formation (in hands and feet), syndesmophytes production and associated HLAB27 antigen are distinguishing features.

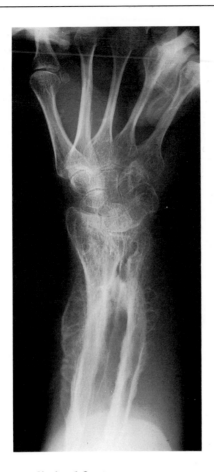

Relevant clinical features

- Blue sclerae with white rings around corneae.
- Multiple deformities of long bones.
- Increasing deafness.

CASE 56

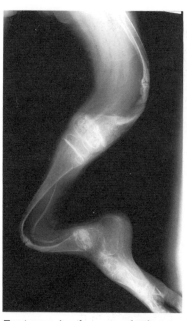

Observations
■ All bones slender, of low density, with thin cortices (osteoporosis).
■ Bowing deformities of radius and ulna due to bone softening, causing multiple fractures which show abundant callus formation.

Features: Another example showing thinning and bowing of femur, tibia and fibula. Ununited fractures midshaft femur and tibia. Note marked osteoporosis.

Diagnosis
OSTEOGENESIS IMPERFECTA: (syn. fragilitas ossium) hereditary deficiency of osteoblasts.

Differential diagnosis
NON-ACCIDENTAL INJURY: bones of normal calibre and density. Deformities only at the site of fractures. Fractures usually metaphyseal.

RICKETS: metaphyses also abnormal (see **Case 39**).

NEUROFIBROMATOSIS: bowing deformities with skin lesions. Associated with pseudofractures. See **Case 100**.

Notes
Autosomal dominant. Two main forms:

■ *Congenital*: the more severe type. May cause still birth. Presents at birth with multiple diaphyseal fractures, thinned and bowed long bones. The skull ossification is defective with wide sutures and wormian bones. May be fatal. Blue sclerae uncommon in neonatal type.

■ *Intermediate*: manifests in puberty or adulthood with deformities, deafness as a result of otosclerosis. Fractures may heal with excess callus. Deformities of the pelvis. Vertebrae show osteoporotic collapse (cod fish type).

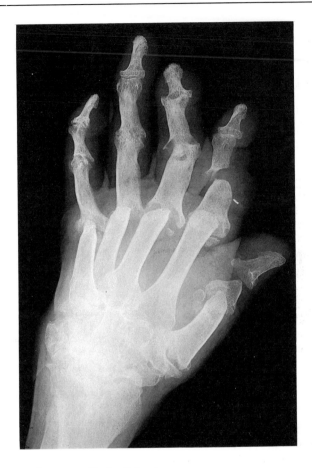

Relevant clinical features

■ Marked deformity of hands and wrists for many years.

■ Telescoping of fingers (main-en-lorgnette).

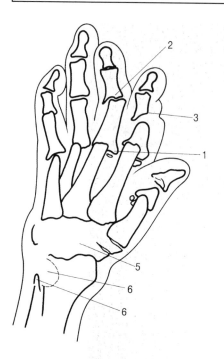

Observations

■ Metacarpal heads worn away leading to shortening of shafts.

■ Flared irregular bases of the proximal phalanges.

■ Similar but less marked changes around PIP joints.

■ Loss of normal alignment at MCP and PIP joints leading to subluxation.

■ Carpal joint spaces reduced and irregular with fusion of several bones.

■ Notching of medial aspect of radius; distal end of ulna tapered and irregular.

Diagnosis

ARTHRITIS MUTILANS: rheumatoid arthritis.

Differential diagnosis

PSORIATIC ARTHROPATHY: DIP joints particularly involved. (See *Case 29*).

Notes

These appearances represent the most advanced stage of joint destruction by rheumatoid arthritis leading to 'telescoping' of the fingers. (Note: DIP joints virtually spared.) Carpal bone ankylosis is a common result. Condition virtually painless presumably due to associated peripheral neuropathy and steroid therapy, both of which may be partially responsible for the joint disorganisation.

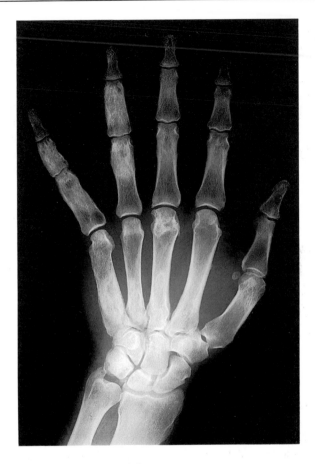

Relevant clinical features
■ Pain and deformity affecting several bones of the hand.

CASE 58

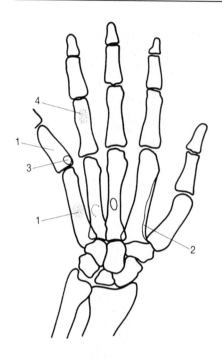

Observations
- Expansion of medullary cavity.
- Cortical thickening.
- Well-defined low-density 'cyst-like' lesions, some that have a sclerotic rim (soap bubble appearance).
- Increased density in medullary region 'ground glass' appearance.

Diagnosis
POLYOSTOTIC FIBROUS DYSPLASIA: primary fibrous bone dysplasia of unknown origin.

Differential diagnosis
PAGET'S DISEASE: some features similar; patient in older age group. (*Case 18*)

Notes
Affected bones soft with deformities and fractures. Low-density lesions may be associated with sclerotic lesions. Can involve single bone, i.e. monostotic. Polyostotic disease has a tendency towards unilateral predominance. Sclerotic involvement of the sphenoid ridge and facial bones causes 'leontiasis ossea'. Nerve compression (optic, auditory, etc.) when skull base involved. Sarcomatous change can occur. Endocrine manifestations include sexual precocity, hyperthyroidism, hyperparathyroidism, gynaecomastia, acceleration of skeletal growth, acromegaly. Female precocious puberty with 'café au lait' skin lesions comprises Albright–McCune syndrome.

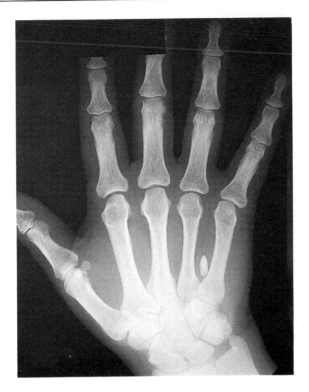

Relevant clinical features

■ Incidental finding.

CASE 59

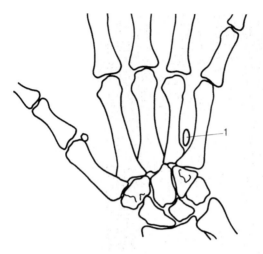

Observations
- Oat-shaped calcification in muscle.

Diagnosis
CYSTICERCOSIS: parasitic infestation.

Notes
Caused by infestation, of tapeworm *Taenia solium*. Cyst stage in muscle dies and calcifies. In 10% 'pin-head' densities on plain skull X-rays, due to calcification of scolex of parasites within brain tissue.

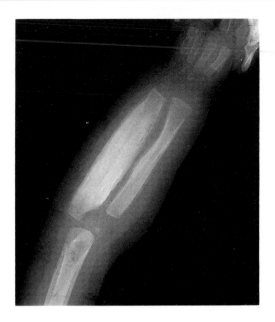

Relevant clinical features

■ Sudden onset of tender soft-tissue swellings over mandibles, clavicles and both arms.

■ Febrile.

CASE 60

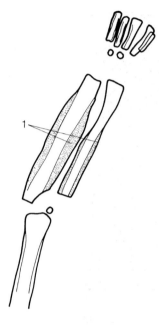

Observations
■ Marked widening of diaphyses of radius and ulna with dense thick cortex.

Diagnosis
INFANTILE CORTICAL HYPEROSTOSIS: (syn. Caffey's syndrome) benign periosteal disease.

Differential diagnosis
NON-ACCIDENTAL INJURY: rarely below age of 6 months. Bruising and metaphyseal fractures common.

HYPERVITAMINOSIS A: usually in child over the age of 2 years.

SYPHILIS: metaphyseal erosion. Metacarpals and phalanges show periosteal reaction.

Notes
Unknown aetiology. Onset almost always under 6 months age. May involve all bones except phalanges. Metaphyses and epiphyses normal. Affects clavicles, mandibles, skull, ulnae and scapulae. Raised ESR and serum phosphatase during acute phase. Usually resolves spontaneously in weeks to a few months. Relapses may occur; rarely becomes chronic.

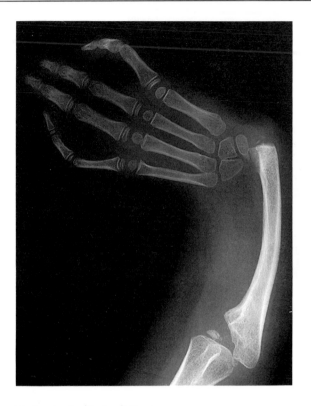

Relevant clinical features

Since birth:

■ Club deformity of one hand.
■ Cardiac murmur.

CASE 61

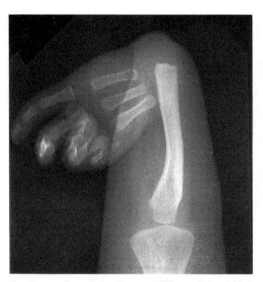

Observations
- Radius absent.
- Ulna curved.
- Thumb absent.

Features: *Complete absence of the radius. Small thumb phalanges present. Features may be associated with thrombocytopenia.*

Diagnosis
RADIAL CLUB HAND: congenital malformation.

Notes
With total absence of the radius, the thumb and radial carpals are also virtually absent. Condition usually sporadic. Associated with a wide range of other congenital abnormalities, particularly cardiac, in this case a VSD. Also seen with the 'VATER' group (i.e. vertebral, anal, tracheo-oesophageal, renal). Bilateral thumb abnormalities (usually triphalangeal), abnormal scaphoids and cardiac defects (ASD) occur in Holt–Oram syndrome. In thrombocytopenia – absent radius syndrome the thumb fingers are usually present (see inset).

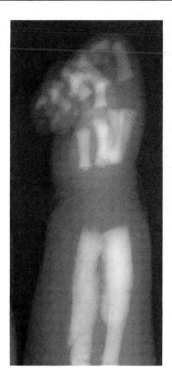

Relevant clinical features

■ Bullae on palms of hands and soles of feet.

■ Saddle deformity of the nose.

CASE 62

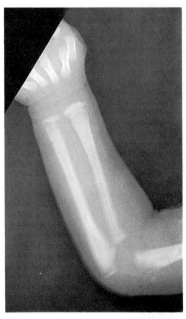

Observations
■ Radius and ulna widened and dense due to irregular new bone formation (florid periostitis).
■ Irregular cupped 'bone ends' – best seen in ulna and metacarpals (due to metaphysitis).
■ Radius has 'bone-within-a-bone' appearance.

Features: Low density transverse metaphyseal bands seen in less severe syphilis.

Diagnosis
CONGENITAL SYPHILIS: granulomatous infection.

Differential diagnosis
Periosteal reactions also seen in INFANTILE CORTICAL HYPEROSTOSIS and healing RICKETS.

Metaphysitis in CONGENITAL RUBELLA and CYTOMEGALOVIRUS INFECTION but usually no periosteal reaction.

Notes
Transplacental infection (after first trimester) leads to widespread symmetrical changes in metaphyses and diaphyses. Curved defects on medial aspects of the tibiae proximally and femorae distally diagnostic of the condition, i.e. Wimberger's sign. Epiphyses not involved.

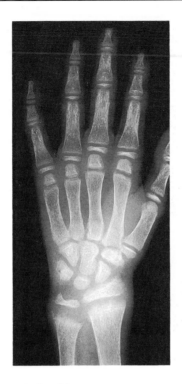

Relevant clinical features

■ Chronic steatorrhoea.

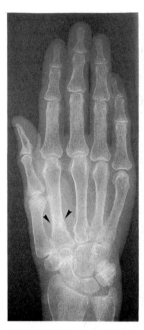

Observations

■ Retarded skeletal development (bone age 10 years).

■ Metaphyseal margins frayed and ill defined (due to poorly calcified bone).

■ Gross metaphyseal cupping (due to weakened bone).

■ Diminished bone density (osteopenia) with thinned cortex and sparse trabecular pattern.

Features: 82 year old malnourished female. No history of trauma. Generalised reduction in bone density with thin cortices due to osteomalacia. Healing Looser's zone base of 2nd metacarpal.

Diagnosis

JUVENILE RICKETS IN COELIAC DISEASE: metabolic bone disease.

Notes

Any cause of vitamin D malabsorption may lead to osteomalacia (or rickets in childhood). Stress fractures occur in weakened bones and the resulting uncalcified osteoid seams (particularly in pelvis, femoral necks, scapulae and ribs) are seen as low-density lines, i.e. Looser's zones (see inset). Weakening of vertebral bodies gives biconcave appearance, i.e. 'cod fish vertebrae'. Associated deformities include bowing of legs, triradiate pelvis and protrusio acetabulae.

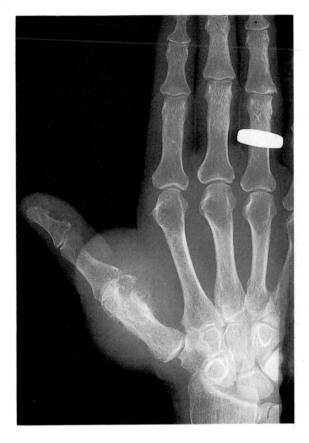

Relevant clinical features
■ Increasing pain and swelling of thenar eminence over 4 weeks.

CASE 64

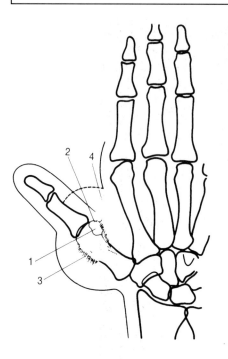

Observations
- Ill-defined low-density lesion in metaphyseal region of first metacarpal.
- Focal destruction of cortex (periarticular osteolysis due to tumour osteoid).
- Spiculated bone arising from cortex at right angles to the shaft, indicating periosteal reaction.
- Large soft-tissue mass with ill-defined densities due to extension of tumour osteoid, which is patchily ossified.

Diagnosis
OSTEOGENIC SARCOMA: (in watch-dial radium paintworker) malignant bone tumour.

Differential diagnosis
OSTEOMYELITIS: often difficult as lamellar periosteal reaction may occur in both.

EWING'S TUMOUR: usually diaphyseal.

Notes
Solitary bone lesion associated with above aggressive radiological features suggests primary bone malignancy. Osteosarcoma is the commonest primary malignant bone tumour. Arises in shaft of long bones. Related to knee joint (50%). Commoner in males in 10–25 year age group. Lung metastases early. Sarcoma may occur in osteochondroma, Paget's disease, fibrous dysplasia, or after exposure to ionising radiation, as in this case.

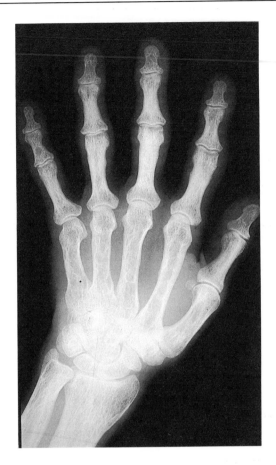

Relevant clinical features

■ Large head.

■ Bowing deformities of lower limbs.

■ Muscular weakness.

CASE 65

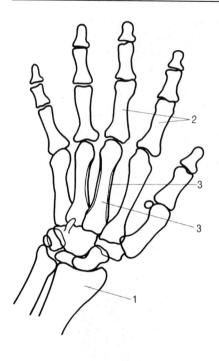

Observations
■ Generalised increased bone density (sclerosis).

■ Phalanges are particularly sclerotic, with obliteration of medullary cavities and thickened trabecular pattern.

■ Metacarpals show thinned cortices and wide medullary cavities.

Diagnosis
HYPERPHOSPHATASIA: (syn. hyperphosphatasemia) primary hereditary bone dysplasia.

Notes
Rare familial failure to produce compact bone. Increased osteoblastic and osteoclastic activity. Raised serum acid and alkaline phosphatase. The fibrous bone is weak, leading to multiple deformities and fractures. The skull vault is generally thickened. The clinical picture of early onset and generalised involvement will differentiate this condition from Paget's disease.

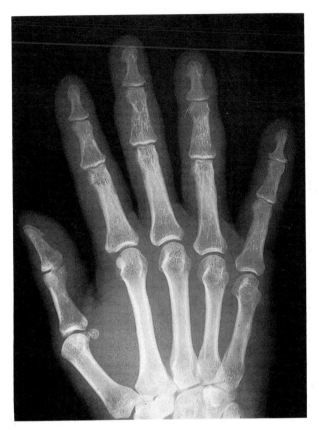

Relevant clinical features
- Progressive shortness of breath.
- Reddish purple rash on hands, feet and face.
- Lymph-node enlargement in neck.

CASE 66

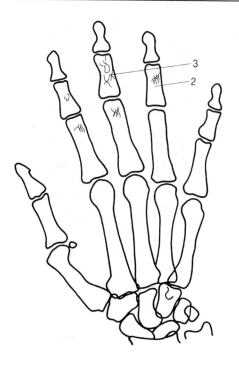

Observations
- Bilateral asymmetrical changes in phalanges.
- Honeycomb trabecular pattern giving lace-like appearance.
- Rounded well-defined low-density lesions in the phalanges (pseudocysts), best seen in intermediate phalanx of third finger.

Diagnosis
SARCOIDOSIS: granulomatous disease of unknown aetiology.

Notes
Bone lesions seen in 5–15% of cases with intrathoracic nodal and pulmonary disease. Commonest in middle, distal phalanges of hand. May involve feet and other bones. Skin lesions (lupus pernio) accompany bone lesions. Absorption of terminal tufts and bone sclerosis may occur. Soft-tissue calcification due to hypercalcaemia in 30% of patients. Commoner in females.

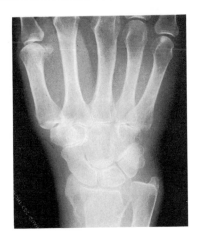 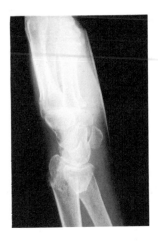

Relevant clinical features

■ Fall on supinated outstretched hand.

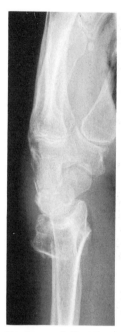

Features: *Colles' fracture demonstrating typical 'dinner fork' deformity.*

Observations
■ Low-density linearities in distal end of radius indicating a comminuted fracture.

■ Volar (palmar, anterior) displacement of distal fragment.

Diagnosis
SMITH'S FRACTURE.

Notes
Fracture uncommon compared with Colles' fracture of the distal radius which is due to falling on an outstretched pronated hand with resulting backward and lateral displacement of the distal fragment.

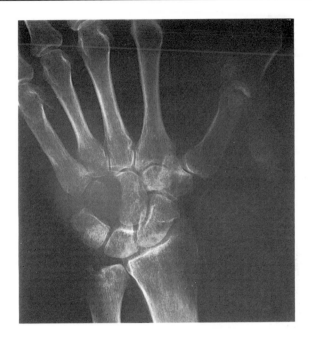

Relevant clinical features
■ Generalised severe bone pain.
■ Loss of weight.

CASE 68

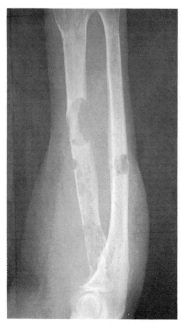

(*Forearm of same patient*)

Observations
- Multiple ill-defined destructive lesions affecting distal radius, ulna and carpal bones.
- Cortices of capitate and hamate destroyed.
- 'Punched out' lesions in opposite forearm.

Diagnosis
MULTIPLE MYELOMA: (plasma cell tumour) malignant primary neoplasm of marrow.

Differential diagnosis
METASTASES: (see *Case 87*).

Notes
Aggressive process causing bone destruction involving multiple bones in an elderly skeleton is usually due to myeloma or metastases. Myelomatosis frequently involves red marrow-containing flat bones of the axial skeleton (skull, spine, ribs, pelvis and proximal long bones). Several different patterns seen. Characteristically punched-out low-density lesions (particularly in the skull vault) without sclerotic margins. But may be just generalised reduced bone density with or without collapse of vertebral bodies – pedicles are spared. Rarely, there may be osteosclerosis. Bone expansion with or without soft-tissue masses commoner in myeloma. Radionuclide bone scan not useful to determine extent of disease, and skeletal radiographic survey is necessary.

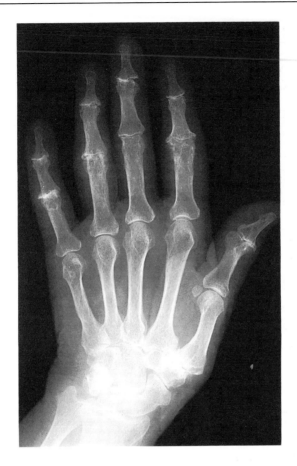

Relevant clinical features

■ Long-standing pain and transient morning stiffness involving fingers of both hands and bases of
thumbs.

■ Hard nodes on dorsum of proximal and distal
interphalangeal joints.

CASE 69

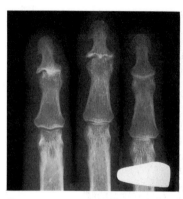

Observations
- *In IP joints*
- Joint space narrowing.
- Bony spurs (osteophytes) at joint margins.
- Well-defined low-density lesions (subarticular cysts).

In CMC joints of thumb
- Increased density (sclerosis) of subchondral bone.

Features: *Irregularity of the articular margins (erosions) affecting distal IP joints, middle ring and little finger.*

Diagnosis
OSTEOARTHROSIS: (syn. osteoarthritis) degenerative joint disease.

Differential diagnosis
PSORIASIS: (see **Case 29**).

RHEUMATOID ARTHRITIS: (see **Case 92**).

Notes
Osteoarthrosis of hand commoner in females and has a familial tendency. Radiographic features:

- Joint space narrowing: due to thinning of cartilage (which may calcify).
- Osteophytes: bony spurs at joint margins due to reactive hyperplasia produces palpable nodes (Heberden's) at DIP joints and at proximal IP joints (Bouchard's). See inset. May detach to form intra-articular loose bodies.
- Sclerosis of subchondral bone: reaction to stress.
- Subarticular cysts: may occur early or late in disease. Small or large, usually with dense rim. Due to traumatic defects in articular cartilage.
- Usually involves large joints (knees and hips) and apophyseal joints of cervical and lumbar spine i.e. those most subjected to stress.
- Spine: apophyseal joints cervical and lumbar region.

Complications: lateral subluxation of femoral head and genu varus deformity of knees. Erosive changes may occur in IP joints due to breakdown of subarticular cysts (see inset).

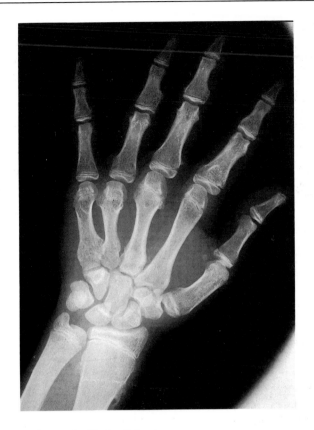

Relevant clinical features
■ Hard painless swellings near joints.

CASE 70

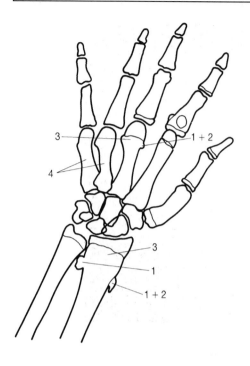

Observations

- Multiple bony protruberances (exostoses) at metaphyses and directed away from joints.
- Best seen in radius and third metacarpal.
- Some metaphyses widened (modelling deformities).
- Short fourth and fifth metacarpals.

Diagnosis

DIAPHYSEAL ACLASIA: (syn. hereditary multiple exostoses, multiple osteochondromata) inherited bone dysplasia.

Notes

Autosomal dominant inheritance. Usually presents in childhood. Often involves several long bones, especially in lower limbs. May cause limb shortening and Madelung's deformity. Membrane bones never involved. May be symptoms due to pressure on nerves, vessels and spinal cord. Bones tend to remodel partially or completely before epiphyseal closure. Cartilage caps may calcify and be seen on radiographs. Chondrosarcomatous change in 10–20%.

CASE 71: Girl aged 3 years

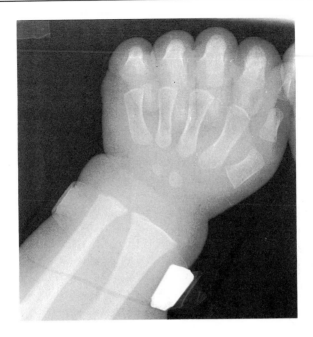

Relevant clinical features
■ Stunted growth and mental retardation.
■ Broad puffy face with large protruberant tongue.
■ Prominent abdomen with umbilical hernia.

CASE 71

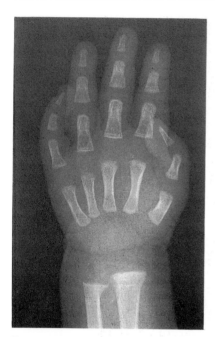

Observations
- Short thick metacarpals.
- Configuration of ossification centres indicates very delayed skeletal maturation (12 months).

Features: Short thick thumb metacarpal. Hypoplastic middle and terminal phalanges 5th finger.

Diagnosis
CRETINISM: metabolic/endocrine disorder.

Notes
Effects of absent thyroid gland not present at birth because of maternal hormones. After birth, skeletal maturation is very slow with delayed appearance of epiphyses, which may be multicentric and leads to dwarfism.

- Skull: wormian bones, wide sutures with delayed closure. Small base. Sinuses small. Dentition delayed.
- Spine and pelvis: anterior spur on lower thoracic and upper lumbar vertebral bodies (like mucopolysaccharidoses) with kyphosis. Narrow pelvis with coxavara.
- Long bones all shortened. Epiphyses may show multicentric ossification, particularly at femoral heads (cf. Perthe's disease, Down's syndrome and multiple epiphyseal dysplasia).
- Tubular bones: metacarpals and little finger phalanges shortened (see inset). Early diagnosis important to prevent mental deficiency. Bone changes regress completely with treatment.

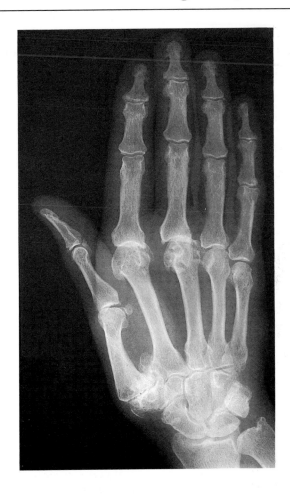

Relevant clinical features
■ Professional knitter.
■ Painful stiff swollen bases of thumbs and knuckles of both hands.

CASE 72

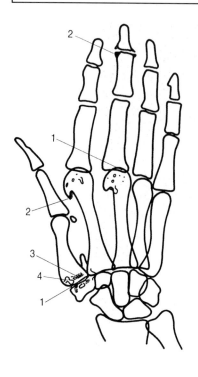

Observations

- Narrowing of joint spaces at CMC joint of thumb and MCP joints of index and middle fingers.
- Bony protruberances (osteophytes) at joint margins.
- Increased density of margins of CMC joint.
- Small ill-defined lucency (subarticular cyst) base of thumb metacarpal.

Diagnosis

OSTEOARTHROSIS: (syn. osteoarthritis) degenerative joint disease.

Notes

This unusual distribution of joint involvement is determined by the repetitive stress at the joints. (Thumb CMC joint is a common site.) Abnormal stress (e.g. from deformity or fracture) may cause osteoarthritis of almost any joint. In above case both hands used in knitting, symmetrical changes seen. For usual distribution and radiographic features of osteoarthrosis see *Case 69*.

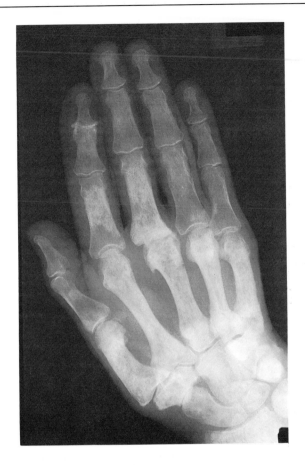

Relevant clinical features
■ Severe generalised bone pain.

CASE 73

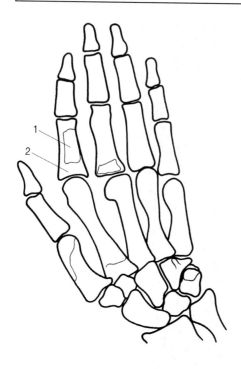

Observations
- Generalised ill-defined patchy areas of increased and decreased bone density (sclerosis and lysis).
- Bone shape and size normal.

Diagnosis
METASTASES FROM PROSTATIC CANCER: secondary malignant bone disease.

Notes
Multiple bones are involved in the above case. Osteoblastic response causes a slower rate of tumour growth, often with resulting hypercalcaemia. This sclerotic and lytic pattern (mixed response) is seen in metastases from carcinoma of prostate, breast (particularly following therapy), pancreas, colon, bladder and lung.

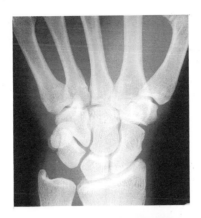

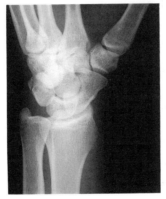

Relevant clinical features

■ Heavy weight fell on dorsum of hand.
■ Tender swelling over ulnar aspect of dorsum.

CASE 74

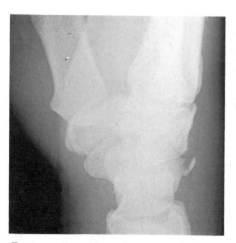

Observations

■ Low-density line in distal part of body of triquetrum.

Features: *Lateral wrist view. The AP film may not show this fracture.*

Diagnosis

FRACTURE OF BODY OF TRIQUETRUM.

Notes

Uncommon fracture site. Much more common is avulsion fracture through the dorsal aspect of the triquetrum (see inset). This is an avulsion injury at the attachment of radio-triquetral and ulnartriquetral ligaments. Triquetral fracture is the second most common carpal bone fracture.

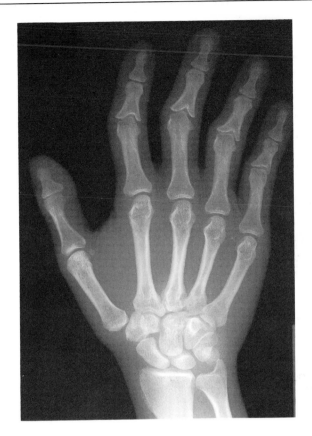

Relevant clinical features
■ Sparse and slow-growing hair.
■ Patchy areas of alopecia.
■ Large bulbous nose.

CASE 75

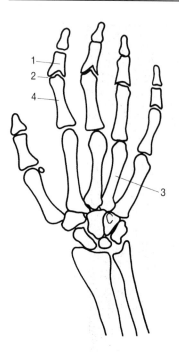

Observations

■ Short intermediate pha-
langes. Their splayed notched
bases indicate that cone-
shaped epiphyses were present.
■ Ulnar deviation at PIP
joints.
■ Metacarpals short.
■ Proximal phalanges long.

Diagnosis

TRICHORHINOPHALANGEAL SYNDROME.

Notes

Autosomal dominant or recessive inherited disorder. Child develops swelling of proximal
interphalangeal joints with ulnar deviation of middle phalanges. Similar changes may
occur in feet. May be shortening of 4th and 5th metacarpals only.

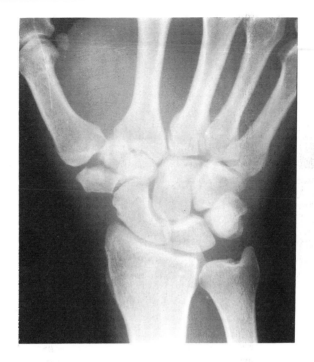

Relevant clinical features

■ Trapped hand.

CASE 76

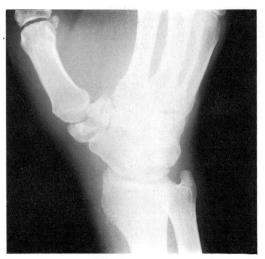

Features: *Oblique projection demonstrating separation of fracture fragments.*

Observations

■ Longitudinal low-density line involving the trapezium and extending to the articular surfaces with separation of the fragments.

Diagnosis

FRACTURE OF TRAPEZIUM.

Notes

Uncommon (5% of all carpal fractures). Due to stress on abducted thumb.

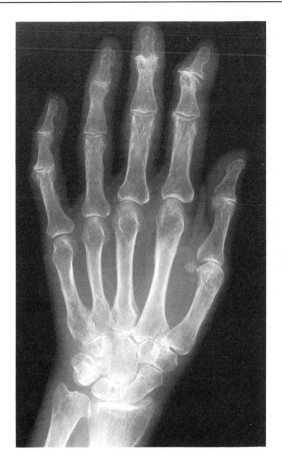

Relevant clinical features
■ Recent hip fracture.
■ Heberden's nodes in index and middle fingers.

CASE 77

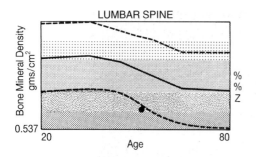

LUMBAR SPINE

Bone Mineral Density gms/cm²

0.537

20   Age   80

%
%
Z

Features: *55 year old woman with long-standing back ache. By comparison with 'age-related mean' this patient's bone density is less than 2 SDs below the mean, consistent with severe postmenopausal osteoporosis.*

Observations

■ Bone density generally reduced (osteopenia).

■ Generalised thinning of bone cortex.

■ Marked osteoarthrosis in DIP joints of index and middle fingers with lateral deviation of terminal phalanx of index finger (see **Case 69**).

Diagnosis

SENILE OSTEOPOROSIS.

Differential diagnosis

Reduced radiographic bone density occurs in:

OSTEOPOROSIS.

OSTEOMALACIA.

PRIMARY HYPERPARATHYROIDISM.

GENERALISED MALIGNANT INFILTRATION.

Notes

Osteoporosis (reduction in mass of normally mineralised bone) commonly occurs in post-menopausal women due to reduced oestrogen levels, leading to fractures, particularly of spine and hip. Difficult to quantify on plain X-ray films but can be measured accurately by dual energy X-ray absorptiometry (DEXA), usually of the lumbar region (see inset).

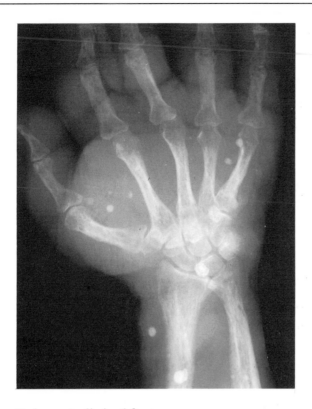

Relevant clinical features
■ Gross lobulated swelling of hand, wrist and forearm.
■ Increasing in size slowly over many years.

CASE 78

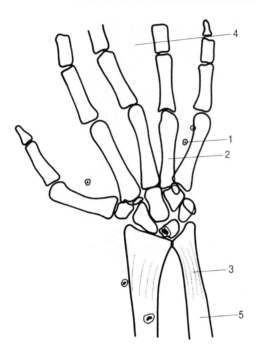

Observations
- Soft-tissue swelling containing multiple small rounded densities with a lucent centre (phleboliths).
- Bones mostly thin and irregular.
- Coarse dense linear pattern in tubular bones in radius and ulna.
- Metacarpals and phalanges spread apart.
- Focal expansion of midshaft of ulna due to bony involvement by the vascular tumour.

Diagnosis
CAVERNOUS HAEMANGIOMA: primary benign vascular tumour of soft tissue origin.

Notes
Haemangiomata contain phleboliths. Adjacent vascular swelling results in pressure atrophy of the bones. Haemangiomata may involve the digit or whole limb. Soft-tissue haemangioma may be associated with numerous enchondromata (Maffucci's syndrome).

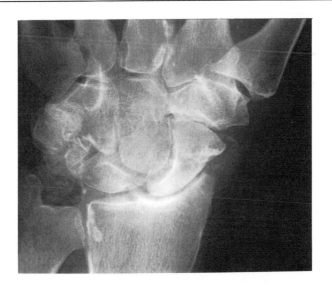

Relevant clinical features

■ Pain and swelling of the wrist for 2 years.
■ No history of trauma.

CASE 79

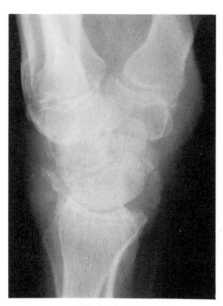

Features: *Osteochondromata well demonstrated on lateral film.*

Observations

■ Multiple small rounded dense opacities closely related to the carpus (calcified and ossified loose bodies in the joint).

■ Radiocarpal joint narrowed with sclerosis of adjacent surfaces (secondary osteoarthrosis).

Diagnosis

SYNOVIAL OSTEOCHONDROMATOSIS: benign synovial neoplasm.

Differential diagnosis

DEGENERATIVE CHANGE: with loose bodies but history of trauma, narrowed joint margins; affects older age group.

NEUROPATHIC JOINT: (see *Case 45*).

Notes

Usually young male adult. Monoarticular involvement often the knee, hip, elbow or shoulder. Synovial metaplasia produces nodules of cartilage which become detached and loose within joint. These grow slowly, calcify and/or ossify. Osteoporosis absent. May lead to secondary degenerative change.

CASE 80: Adult male

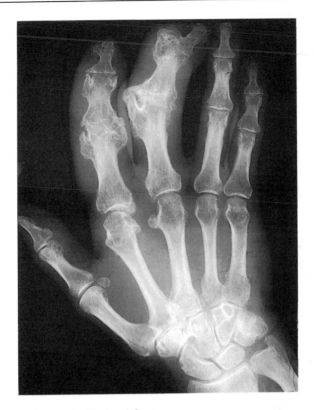

Relevant clinical features

■ Gradual enlargement of index and middle fingers of left hand since childhood.

■ Bony protuberances around joints of these fingers.

■ Soft-tissue swelling of fingers.

CASE 80

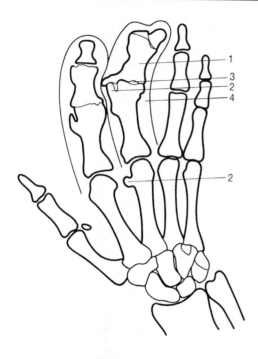

Observations
- Enlarged phalanges.
- Deformities produced by multiple osteochondromata.
- Narrow joint spaces, indicating degenerative changes.
- Soft-tissue thickening due to fatty masses.

Diagnosis
MACRODYSTROPHIA LIPOMATOSA: rare congenital localised disturbance of growth.

Notes
Overgrowth of bone (sometimes with osteochondromata (see *Case 23*) and soft tissues, predominantly the fat. Usually involves the phalanges of one or more fingers. May occur in toes, arm or whole limb.

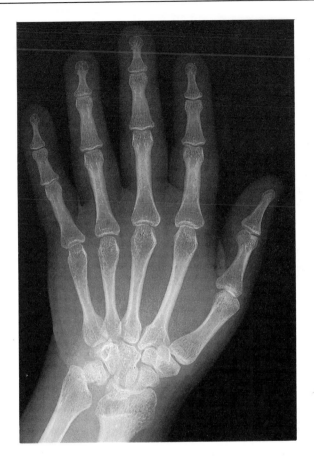

Relevant clinical features

■ Primary amenorrhoea. Very small breasts.

■ Short stature, webbed neck, cubitus valgus deformity.

CASE 81

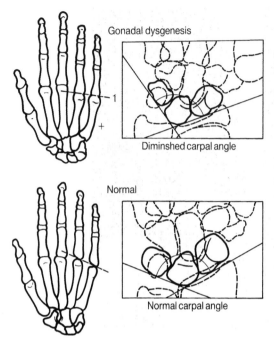

Gonadal dysgenesis

Diminshed carpal angle

Normal

Normal carpal angle

Observations
■ Small hand with shortened metacarpal of ring finger.
■ Carpal angle below normal.
■ Madelung's deformity (see **Case 50**).
■ Reduced bone width and density with thin cortices (indicates osteoporosis and poor modelling due to oestrogen deficiency): best seen in distal phalanges, giving drumstick appearance.

Diagnosis
GONADAL DYSGENESIS: (syn. Turner's syndrome) karotype XO.

Notes
In classical Turner's syndrome (XO) the patient is short, with webbed neck, broad chest, wide separation of nipples, and low posterior hair line. Laparoscopic examination shows streak ovaries. Widespread skeletal abnormalities: retarded maturation, osteoporosis, Madelung's deformity, cubitus valgus and exostosis on medial tibial plateau. Renal and cardiac abnormalities include aortic coarctation and stenosis. May be minimal abnormalities if mosaicism (XO/XX).

Inset

■ Metacarpal line: in Turner's syndrome a line drawn cutting the distal ends of the 4th and 5th metacarpals intersects the 3rd metacarpal (positive sign).
■ Carpal angle: the normal angle is approx. 131°. In Turner's syndrome the angle is reduced.

CASE 82: Adult male

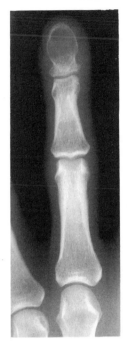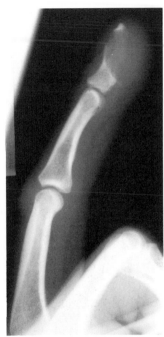

Relevant clinical features
- Penetrating injury to phalanx years ago.
- Increasing swelling since.

CASE 82

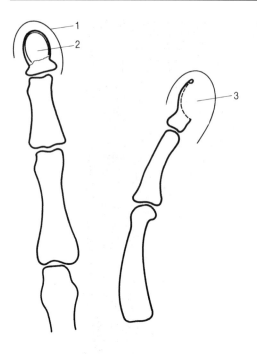

Observations
- Pulp swollen.
- Terminal phalanx expanded by low-density lesion with high-density rim.
- Volar cortex destroyed.

Diagnosis
EPIDERMOID INCLUSION CYST: (syn. implantation dermoid).

Differential diagnosis
ENCHONDROMA: calcification usual (see **Case 17**).

GLOMUS TUMOUR: bluish mass visible clinically.

ANEURYSMAL BONE CYST: metaphyseal in location and before epiphyseal fusion. Rarely in hand.

Notes
Epiphethial tissue driven into bone grows slowly and causes local expansion and replacement of bone.

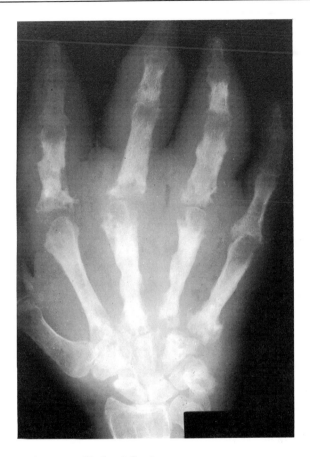

Relevant clinical features
■ Painless swollen foot and hand for 2 years.
■ Several sinuses discharging through the skin.

CASE 83

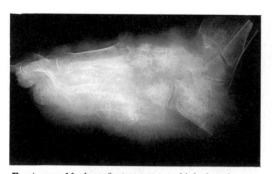

Features: *Madura foot: associated lobulated soft tissue swelling. Destruction of tarsal and metatarsal bones with increased bone density and new bone formation.*

Observations

■ Diffuse lobulated soft-tissue swelling.

■ Well-defined defects (pressure erosion) in the cortex of the tubular bones particularly the ring, and middle fingers and carpal bones.

■ Patchy increase in bone density (sclerosis) and areas of ill-defined low density (bone destruction) indicate spread of soft-tissue infection to bone.

Diagnosis

MYCETOMA: primary soft-tissue fungal infection involving bone.

Notes

Condition due to maduramycetoma or actinomycetes usually seen in hot dry climates (e.g. India, Africa, South America) and affecting the foot, 'Madura foot' (see inset). Infection is from the soil whilst walking barefoot and produces discharging sinuses. May spread to involve the bone, giving bone destruction and periosteal reaction.

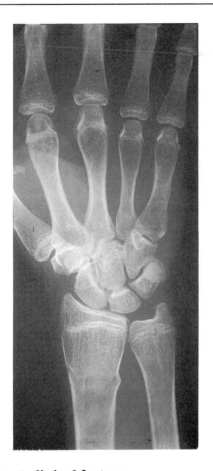

Relevant clinical features
- Injury to wrist.
- Small stature.
- Sexually underdeveloped.

CASE 84

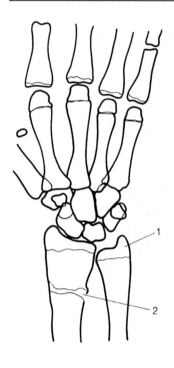

Observations
■ Epiphyses not fused, i.e. skeletal maturation delayed (bone age 16 years).
■ Deformity of trabecular pattern distal radius, with break in the cortex.

Diagnosis
HYPOPITUITARISM: with Colles' fracture. Metabolic/Endocrine disorder and associated trauma.

Notes
Hypopituitary dwarf (Lorraine–Levi type) will have an enlarged or eroded sella turcica if a pituitary tumour (e.g. chromophobe adenoma) is the cause. Normal at birth. Then growth and skeletal maturation and puberty are delayed.

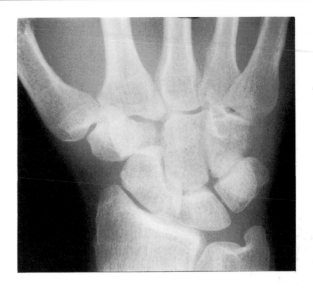

Relevant clinical features

■ Fell off bicycle, landed on wrist.

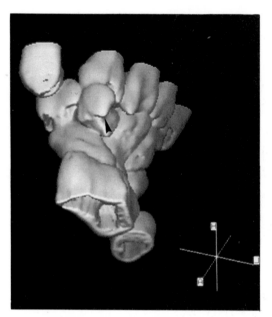

Features: *Clearly shows dorsal displacement of the trapezoid.*

Observations

PA film
■ Trapezoid and trapezium partially superimposed.

CT scan
■ Low-density band through proximal pole of trapezoid indicates fracture line. Dorsal displacement of distal fragment.

Diagnosis

FRACTURE DISLOCATION OF THE TRAPEZOID.

Notes

Unusual injury. Dorsal dislocation occurs due to the wedge shape of the trapezoid. Rarely able to diagnose on plain films, and CT scans required for proper evaluation of any complex fractures in the wrist joint. (Fractures, dislocations and free fragments can be identified readily.)

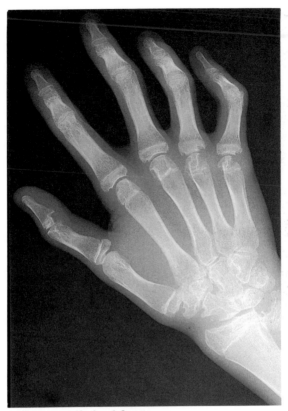

Relevant clinical features

■ Developed low-grade fever 3 years ago.

■ Firm non-tender nodules over extensor surfaces of forearms.

■ Recently swollen stiff painful fingers and left knee.

CASE 86

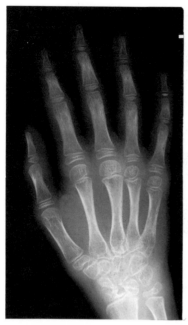

Features: *Systemic onset JCA. 9 year old girl. Soft tissue swelling MCP joints and juxta-articular osteoporosis. Erosions confined to radiocarpal joint.*

Observations

- Low-density bone around joints (juxta-articular osteoporosis) due to disuse and hyperaemia.
- Soft-tissue swelling around MCP joints.
- Reduction in space and marginal defects (erosions) of carpal and MCP joints, due to cartilage erosion and eroding synovial pannus.
- Apparent duplication of cortex (periosteal thickening) affecting several metacarpals and proximal phalanges.
- Premature fusion of epiphyses due to hyperaemia.

Diagnosis

JUVENILE CHRONIC ARTHRITIS (JCA): Rheumatoid factor positive polyarthropathy.

Notes

Several subgroups of JCA exist distinguished by age of onset, articular and extra-articular manifestation, certain serological findings, including rheumatoid factor, anti-nuclear factor and HLAB27 antigen.

- Rheumatoid factor positive polyarthropathy: onset late childhood. Severe arthritis in more than 50% of patients. Erosive polyarthropathy resembles adult type but with periosteal new bone. Cervical spine and large joints more commonly involved. Poor prognosis. RF 100%, ANF 75% (as in this case).
- Systemic onset JCA: pericarditis, myocarditis, anaemia, fever arthralgia, myalgia and hepatosplenomegaly. (RF, ANF negative.) (See inset.) Progressive arthritis 10–25%.
- Large joint arthritis – type 1: early childhood involves large joints (hips and sacroiliac joints spared). Few constitutional symptoms. Chronic iridocyclitis in 50%. (RF negative, ANF 50%.)
- Large joint arthritis – type 2: late childhood. Young boys. Hip and sacroiliac involvement common. Ankylosing spondylitis at follow-up. (HLAB27 positive.)

172

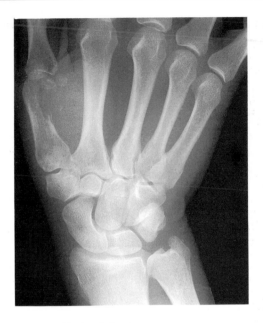

Relevant clinical features
- Painful swollen thenar eminence.
- Heavy smoker.

CASE 87

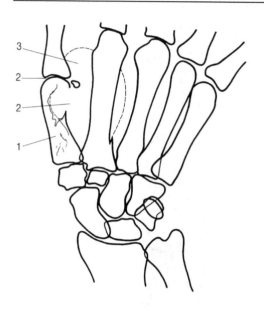

Observations

- Ill-defined, low-density poorly marginated lesion of thumb metacarpal due to tumour in medullary cavity.
- Cortex of bone destroyed medially, but destructive process does not cross the joint.
- Soft-tissue swelling.

Diagnosis

METASTASIS: secondary neoplasm from bronchial carcinoma.

Differential diagnosis

MYELOMA: (see *Case 68*).

Notes

Usually occur in red marrow-containing bones. Pathological fractures common and destructive process *frequently involves the vertebral pedicles* (cf. myeloma). In the axial skeleton, soft-tissue swelling uncommon with metastases, but may occur with myeloma or plasmacytoma. In peripheral skeleton soft-tissue swelling occurs with both. As multiple bones are usually involved in metastatic disease, radionuclide bone scanning, which is more sensitive than radiography, is necessary to determine extent of disease.

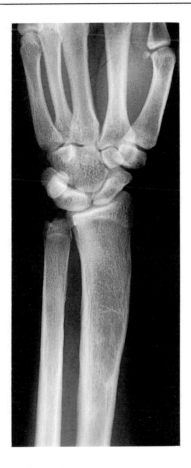

Relevant clinical features

■ For 3 years, weakness, fatigue, weight loss.

■ Patchy yellow/brown skin pigmentation with ecchymoses.

■ Now complaining of pains in the bones.

CASE 88

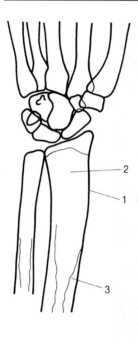

Observations
■ Expanded distal diaphyses and metaphyses of radius and ulna: called Erlenmeyer flask deformity (due to infiltration by Gaucher's cells).

■ Reduced bone density associated with thinning of the cortex.

■ More proximally, cortical thickening of diaphyses due to periosteal reaction.

Diagnosis
GAUCHER'S DISEASE: histiocytic proliferation with lipid deposits.

Differential diagnosis
THALASSAEMIA MAJOR: bone expansion due to marrow hyperplasia. Bone infarction not present. (See *Case 42*).

Notes
Chronic hereditary disorder. Commoner in Jews. Bone marrow, liver and spleen infiltrated by kerasin-containing large reticulum cells, i.e. Gaucher's cells. Commonly involves femora, hips, spine and shoulders. Usually presents with splenomegaly, anaemia and ischaemic necrosis of the femoral and humeral heads due to infarction. Erlenmeyer flask contour commonest in femora. Fractures common. Rare severe infantile form often involves the CNS and respiratory system resulting in death during infancy. Part of a widespread group of diseases including Hand–Schuller–Christian complex consisting of Letterer–Siwe disease and eosinophilic granuloma.

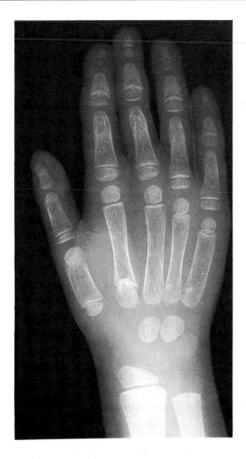

Relevant clinical features
- Large head with small face.
- Drooping shoulders.

CASE 89

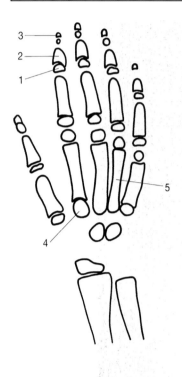

Observations

■ Cone-shaped epiphyses indent metaphyses of the intermediate phalanges of the index to little fingers.

■ Intermediate phalanges are short.

■ Terminal phalanges are hypoplastic.

■ Supernumerary epiphyses at the proximal end of the index metacarpal and also the ring and little finger where they are partially fused.

■ Reduced bone density indicates osteoporosis.

Diagnosis

CLEIDOCRANIAL DYSOSTOSIS: congenital hereditary defect in bone formation.

Notes

Autosomal dominant inheritance. Defect is most marked in ossification of intramembraneous bones mainly of midline structures, but formation of some enchondral bones also faulty.

■ Skull: brachycephalic, wormian bones with wide sutures and fontanelles which close late. Facial bones and sinuses small. Delayed or defective dentition. Mandibles normal.

■ Thorax: clavicles absent or hypoplastic. Unfused vertebral neural arches, narrow thorax. Supernumerary ribs.

■ Pelvis: delayed or absent ossification of bones forming symphysis pubis. Coxavara from deformed femoral necks.

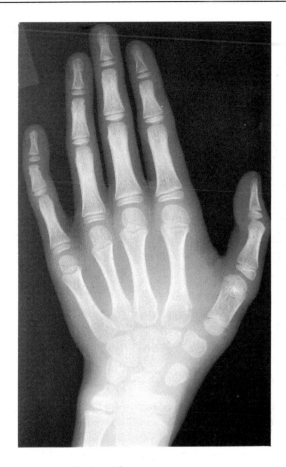

Relevant clinical features

■ Short thumbs and short great toes noted at birth.

■ Since age 5 years developed soft-tissue swellings in neck and over back of thorax. These now feel hard.

CASE 90

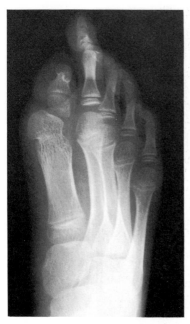

Features: *Short great toe due to hypoplastic proximal phalanx. Metatarsal head deformed.*

Observations
■ Thumb metacarpal short with supernumerary epiphysis distally.

■ Little finger curved due to asymmetrical shortening of middle phalanx, i.e. clinodactyly.

Diagnosis
MYOSITIS OSSIFICANS PROGRESSIVA: (syn. fibrodysplasia ossificans progressiva) congenital hereditary disorder of connective tissues. Unknown cause.

Notes
Characteristic short thumbs and short great toes allowing diagnosis at birth. In the first decade, inflammatory foci appear in tendons, ligaments and fascia. Later these ossify progressively producing crippling deformities with loss of function and ankylosis of joints. Course variable.

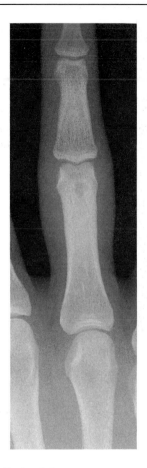

Relevant clinical features

■ For past 12 months increasing soft-tissue swelling over palmar aspect of middle finger near to PIP joint.

■ Slightly painful over past 2 months.

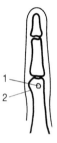

1
2

Observations
■ Small oval well-defined low-density lesion in head of proximal phalanx of middle finger. Margins are dense, i.e. lesion is corticated.

■ Associated soft-tissue swelling.

Diagnosis
PIGMENTED VILLONODULAR SYNOVITIS: of tendon sheath; benign tumour of synovium.

Differential diagnosis
OSTEOID OSTEOMA: (see *Case 22*).

BRODIES ABSESS.

Notes
Usually in young adults. Most commonly arises in synovium of large joints, particularly the knee. May occur in tendon sheath of feet or hands.

■ In joint PVNS: marked soft-tissue swelling due to effusion and synovial mass. Later corticated para-articular erosions appear, enlarge and typically involve both sides of the joint. No osteoporosis.

■ In tendon sheath PVNS: may be only soft-tissue swelling which may be distant from joint. In 25% of cases, intraosseous extension produces a corticated defect in adjacent bone (as in this case).

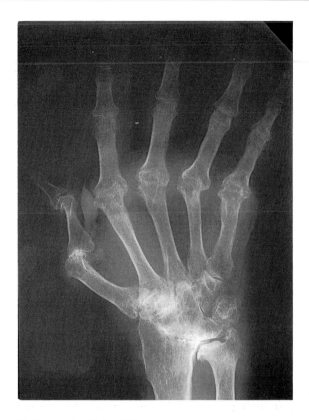

Relevant clinical features

■ Many years of pain, swelling, stiffness of both hands and wrist.

■ Now deformed fingers and thumbs.

CASE 92

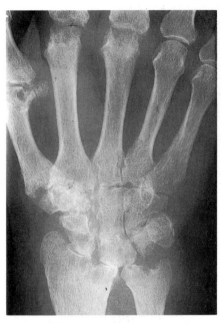

Observations
■ Bony ankylosis of carpal bones and radiocarpal joint.
■ Subluxation and ulnar deviation of fingers.
■ Adduction deformity of thumb.

Features: *Marked erosive changes of wrist carpal bones. These changes precede bony and fibrous ankylosis.*

Diagnosis
RHEUMATOID ARTHRITIS: severe chronic type.

Differential diagnosis
LIPOIDERMATOARTHRITIS: cutaneous soft-tissue nodes with destructive polyarthropathy, affecting PIP joints.

Notes
Radiographic features (notes refer to both **Case 3** and **Case 92**):

■ Erosions: (see inset) 'en face' have a cyst-like appearance. With healing may develop dense peripheries, i.e. 'corticated'. Erosions may spread to form subarticular cyst-like lesions 'geodes'.
■ Joint space narrowing: develops due to cartilage destruction.
■ Juxta-articular osteoporosis: results from hyperaemia and disuse.

Patterns of involvement: Variable, may involve knees (causes Baker's cyst), hips (protrusioacetabulae), cervical spine (atlantoaxial joint and facet joints).

Complications: subluxations; deformities (swan-neck and boutoniere of fingers, fibrous and bony ankylosis especially of wrist, arthritis mutilans (see **Case 57**); degenerative changes, septic arthritis; (particularly with steroid therapy), secondary amyloidosis.

Extraosseous radiographic changes: lungs – pleural effusions, fibrosing alveolitis, necrobiotic nodules, Caplan's syndrome, obliterative bronchiolitis. Heart – pericardial effusions, pericarditis, valvulitis.

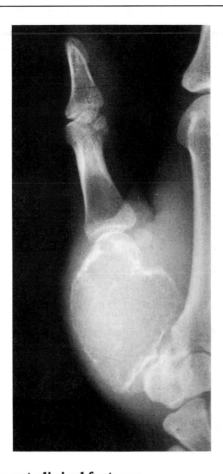

Relevant clinical features

■ Six-week history of pain and progressive swelling at the base of the thumb.

CASE 93

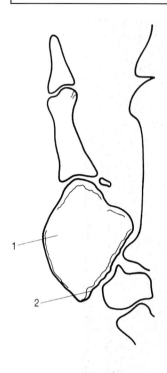

Observations
■ Eccentric low-density expansile lesion affecting the base and shaft of the thumb metacarpal associated with cortical thinning.
■ Extension to the articular margin.

Diagnosis
ANEURYSMAL BONE CYST: primary benign bone tumour.

Differential diagnosis
GIANT CELL TUMOUR: (see **Case 49**).

FIBROUS DYSPLASIA: (see **Case 58**).

METASTASES AND PLASMA CYTOMA: (see **Case 87** and **Case 68**).

Notes
Majority occur in the immature skeleton. Usually involves metaphyses of long bones, pelvis or vertebrae. If the lesion extends into the epiphysis it resembles a giant cell tumour (as in the above case). Fractures may occur. If vertebrae involved cord compression and neurological symptoms sometimes occur.

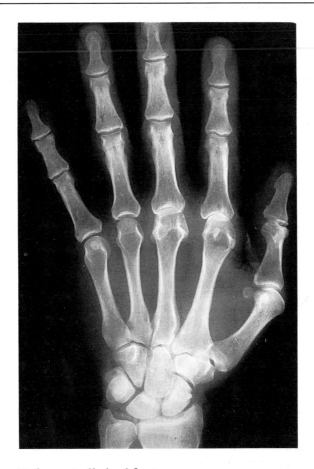

Relevant clinical features

- Painful right wrist.
- Greyish pigmentation to skin.
- Enlarged liver.

CASE 94

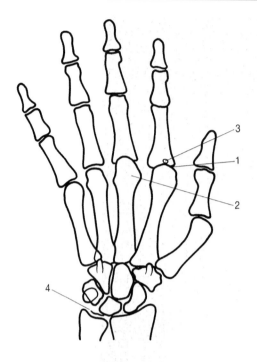

Observations
■ Narrowing of MCP joint spaces of index and middle fingers.
■ These metacarpal heads are widened.
■ Subarticular cyst in proximal phalanx of index finger.
■ Calcification of cartilage over head of radius and ulna (chondrocalcinosis).

Diagnosis
PRIMARY HAEMOCHROMATOSIS: (syn. bronzed diabetes).

Notes
Inherited defect allowing excessive iron absorption and widespread deposition of iron within tissues including synovium. This inhibits pyrophosphate activity and leads to deposition of calcium pyrophosphate in cartilage leading to premature osteoarthrosis. Much more common in middle-aged men. Skeletal involvement diagnosed by combination of:

■ Premature degenerative changes: in MCP joints of index and middle fingers (may be similar changes in wrists, knees and hips).
■ Chondrocalcinosis: may be widespread, including menisci and symphysis pubis.
■ Osteoporosis.

Deposition of iron in skin, pancreas, liver, spleen and testes produces bronzed skin, diabetes, cirrhosis and testicular atrophy. Other causes of chondrocalcinosis are: osteoarthrosis, gout, pyrophosphate arthropathy, psoriatic arthritis, rheumatoid arthritis and ochronosis.

CASE 95: Adult female from Kenya

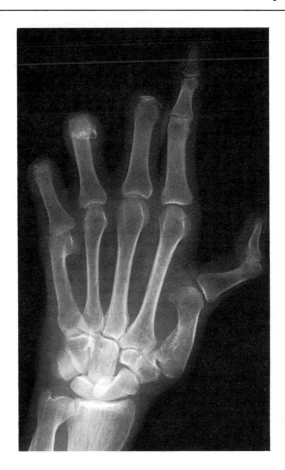

Relevant clinical features

■ Long-standing impaired sensation in both hands.

■ Claw left hand with ulceration of the fingers.

■ Hypopigmented macules for many years on lateral aspects of arms and legs.

CASE 95

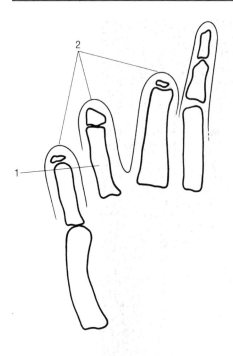

Observations
■ Generalised loss in bone density (osteoporosis).
■ Absorption of terminal phalanges, of middle, ring and little finger.

Diagnosis
TUBERCULOID LEPROSY: with neuropathic change; primary bone infection.

Differential diagnosis
SYRINGOMYELIA.

CONGENITAL INSENSITIVITY TO PAIN.

Notes
Three distinct types of bone lesions: tuberculoid, lepromatous and mixed. In the more common neuropathic form there is progressive resorption of bone due to nerve involvement, superimposed trauma and infection beginning in the distal phalanges of the hand. Bone destruction also occurs in the legs, feet and nasal bones.

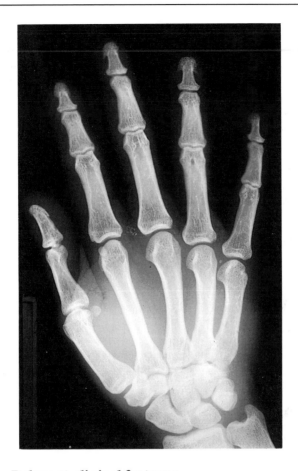

Relevant clinical features
■ Soft-tissue swelling between index and middle fingers of right hand.

CASE 96

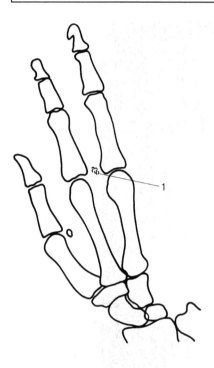

Observations
■ Serpiginous beaded density in soft tissues between proximal phalanges of index and middle fingers due to subcutaneous calcified dead parasite.

Diagnosis
FILARIASIS: parasitic soft-tissue infestation.

Notes
Filariasis: tropical infection with certain worms, i.e. *Wucheria bancrofti, Brugia malayi, Loa Loa, Onchocerca volvulus*. Fine filiform worms lie coiled in lymphatics. Some die and calcify. More common in lower limbs. Transmission via mosquitos and other vectors. Repeated infections lead to elephantiasis (cf. cysticercosis (**Case 59**)).

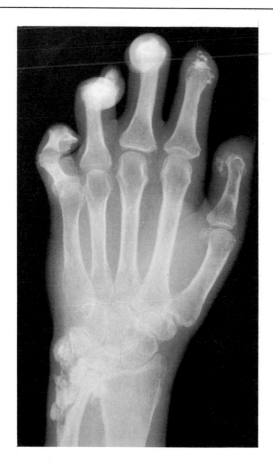

Relevant clinical features
- Raynaud's phenomenon for many years.
- Soft tissues of fingers atrophic.
- Skin ulcerated.
- Flexion deformity of fingers.

CASE 97

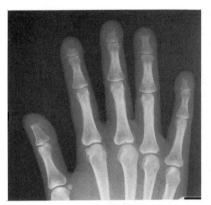

Features: *Loss of terminal tips. Acro-osteolysis; often the earliest bone changes.*

Observations

■ Loss of terminal phalanx of thumb and index finger.

■ Generalised thinning of soft tissue with flexion contractures of the fingers.

■ Calcification in soft tissues around DIP joint of thumb and index finger and wrist, i.e. periarticular in distribution.

■ Reduced bone density due to disuse.

Diagnosis

SCLERODERMA: collagen vascular disease.

Notes

Multiorgan chronic disorder. Raynaud's phenomenon associated with vasospastic and occlusive changes in digital arteries. Commoner in hands than in feet. In 60% leads to resorption of distal phalangeal tufts (see inset). Soft-tissue atrophy associated with calcific deposits. Joint symptoms are frequent with periarticular swelling and osteoporosis. Erosions similar to rheumatoid arthritis may also infrequently develop. Gastrointestinal involvement in 50%, especially atonic, and dilated oesophagus. Interstitial fibrotic lung disease in 25%. Heart involvement with cardiomyopathy in 35%.

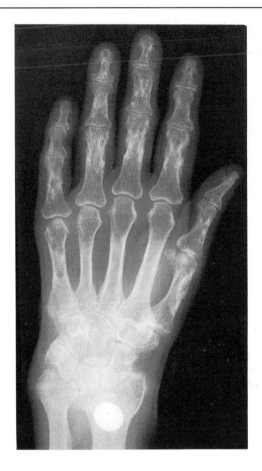

Relevant clinical features
- Mentally retarded and epileptic.
- Adenoma sebaceum on face.

CASE 98

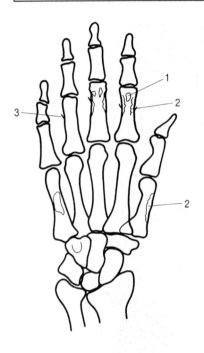

Observations
■ Multiple well-defined areas of reduced density (cyst-like) in tubular bones.
■ Cortical and trabecular thickening in phalanges and thumb metacarpal.
■ Cortical spurs at tendinous insertions.

Diagnosis
TUBEROUS SCLEROSIS: inherited defective development of ectodermal tissues.

Notes
Condition characterised by multiple hamartomatous lesions in brain, skeletal system, kidneys and lungs. Skeletal changes described above in the hands are virtually pathognomonic. Areas of increased density may occur in other bones (e.g. flame-shaped opacities in ilia). Calcified periventricular nodules seen on skull X-ray or CT head scan. Subungual defects, 'café-au-lait' spots seen. Associated hamartomatous tumours include angiomyolipomas of kidney and retinal phakomas.

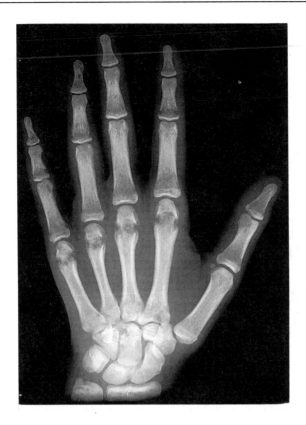

Relevant clinical features

■ Febrile and toxic.

■ Swollen and painful joints of hand.

■ Multiple bruises.

CASE 99

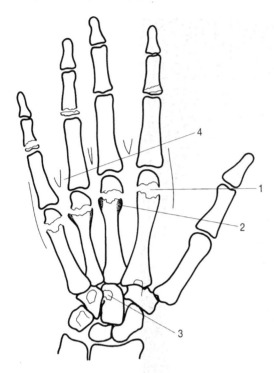

Observations
- Irregular low-density bands across metaphyses, particularly in metacarpals.
- Thickening of cortices involving adjacent diaphyses (periosteal reaction).
- Ill-defined low-density area in capitate (lytic lesion).
- Associated soft-tissue swelling.

Diagnosis
ACUTE LEUKAEMIA: primary malignant marrow tumour.

Differential diagnosis
ROUND CELL TUMOURS: (neuroblastoma and malignant histiocytosis) marrow cytology, blood and urine biochemistry will differentiate.

SCURVY AND SYPHILIS: metaphyseal bands under the age of 2 years.

Notes
Commonest in 2–5 years age group. Widespread skeletal involvement in 50%. Malignant marrow cells inhibit bone formation, destroy existing bone, and may infiltrate the synovium. Earliest lesions are low-density transverse metaphyseal bands. Periosteal new bone is due to cortical infiltration. May be associated with generalised reduction in bone density (osteoporosis) and destructive low-density (lytic) lesions. If meningeal involvement, raised intracranial pressure may lead to spread of cranial sutures. Predisposing factors include exposure to ionising radiation, Down's syndrome, osteopetrosis and bilateral agenesis of radii.

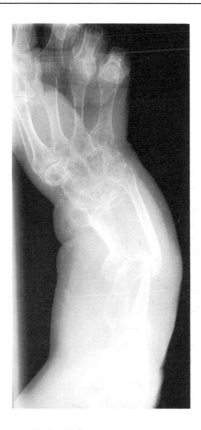

Relevant clinical features

■ 'Café-au-lait' spots.

■ Shortened and deformed right forearm.

CASE 100

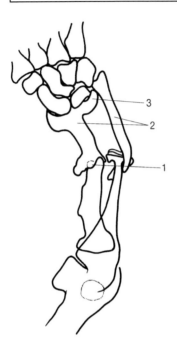

Observations
- Pseudoarthrosis of radius and ulna.
- Deformed short radius and ulna.
- Reduced density of all bones with thinned cortices (osteoporosis).

Diagnosis
NEUROFIBROMATOSIS: hereditary defective development of mesodermal and neuroectodermal tissues (syn. Von Recklinghausen's disease).

Notes
Neurofibromatosis primarily involves the skin (fibromata, naevi and areas of pigmentation) and nervous system (fibromata in peripheral and cranial nerves). Pseudoarthrosis is a rare condition; it may precede skin changes by several years and may not be associated with other neurofibromatous bone lesions. Neurofibromatosis may cause:

- Abnormalities in bone development: absent orbital plates or sphenoid wing, ribbon deformities of ribs, spina bifida, pes cavus, club foot.
- Pressure effects from tumours: scalloped vertebral bodies, enlarged intervertebral foramina, rib notching.
- Intraosseous infiltration: widening, overgrowth or undergrowth of bones.

Other associations: endocrine tumours, phaeochromocytoma, intrathoracic meningocele, menigioma, glioma, aortic coarctation, renal artery stenosis.

Index

Index